The Quiet Earth

Thirteen Essays on the Interrelationship
Between Nature and Human Health

Edited by: John Hanson Mitchell
Illustrated by: Barry Van Dusen

Published by the
Massachusetts Audubon Society
Lincoln, MA 01773

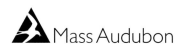
Mass Audubon

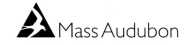

Published by the
Massachusetts Audubon Society as a benefit of membership, 2016

Copyright 2016 by the Massachusetts Audubon Society
ISBN 978-0-9863869-2-3

Editor: John Hanson Mitchell
Artist: Barry Van Dusen
Copyeditor: Ann Prince
Production Manager: Rose Murphy
Designer: Lynne Foy
Poetry Editors: Susan Richmond and Wendy Drexler
Proofreaders: Janet Foster, Betty Graham

Mass Audubon works to protect the nature of Massachusetts for people and wildlife. Together with more than 100,000 members, we care for 35,000 acres of conservation land; provide school, camp, and other educational programs for 225,000 children and adults annually; and advocate for sound environmental policies at local, state, and federal levels. Founded in 1896 by two inspirational women who were committed to the protection of birds, Mass Audubon is now one of the largest and most prominent conservation organizations in New England. Today we are respected for our sound science, successful advocacy, and innovative approaches to connecting people and nature. Each year, our statewide network of wildlife sanctuaries welcomes nearly half a million visitors of all ages, abilities, and backgrounds and serves as the base for our work. To support these important efforts, call 800-AUDUBON (800-283-8266) or visit www.massaudubon.org.

The Quiet Earth is part of a book series produced each year as a Mass Audubon premium. To learn more visit www.massaudubon.org

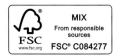

Table of Contents

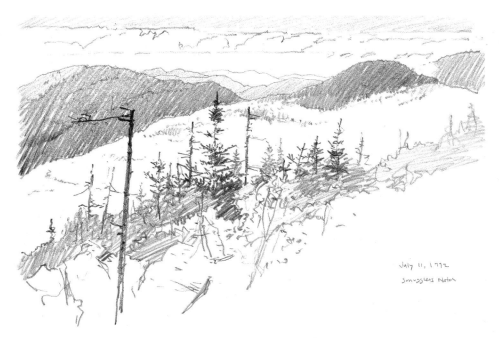

July 11, 1992
Smugglers Notch

Shaking Off the Snow

by Jeffrey Harrison

The snow was heavy and clung thickly to the trees,
and there was no sun yet to start it melting
and give them some relief. Some trees had cracked,
others bowed in fringed arcs over the trail,
and some bent so low they blocked the trail entirely.
I shook one off and watched it spring back up
and laughed as it dumped snow on me,
and on the snow-covered ground with muffled thunder.

Then I kept following the closed-in trail
and opening it up, shaking the trees
and letting them go, and showering myself with snow.
The branches that sometimes whipped me in the face

and the clumps of snow stinging my neck and forehead
were a price worth paying to see the trees fly up.
One pulled my glove right off, a woolen leaf.
One good-sized oak almost lifted me off the ground.

I thought of Frost's birches, lifting the boy up,
and of his crow that shook snow down on him,
changing his mood. It seemed I needed more
than just a dusting. I needed to be covered
from head to toe. And I couldn't get enough
of the bowed-over trees springing back up.
By the end, I was soaked, sweating under my clothes,
almost happy, my pockets filled with snow.

From *Into Daylight* (Tupelo Press 2014)

Preface

Green Health

On his first ascent of Mount Katahdin in 1846, Henry Thoreau looked out over the savage, inhuman vistas of wilderness and was shocked by the vast indifference of the world below him. "Think of our life in nature," he wrote about the event. "…to come in contact with it—rocks, trees, wind on our cheeks! The solid earth! the actual world! the common sense! Contact! Contact! Who are we? Where are we?"

Fifty years later, in 1896, on the Pacific Island of Tahiti, the artist Paul Gauguin, confronted with what he viewed as the savage, free aspect of the native people, had a vaguely similar reaction. He created a painting of a group of native Tahitians each looking in a different direction and titled it: *"Where Do We Come From? Who Are We? Where Are We Going?"*

These are good questions. It may seem hard to believe, passing through a busy airport, or immersed in the turmoil of city streets that we, the multitudes, are in fact merely Cro-Magnon hunter-gatherers only recently emerged from the wide savannahs of the Serengeti Plain of Africa. But the fact is, we are deeply ensconced in the natural world, even though we may not realize it. You have but to watch some tight-vested urbane banker striding along a city street tear open a stubborn plastic-wrapped bag of peanuts with his teeth to understand this. Or to reach even farther back on our evolutionary tree, all you have to do is watch a group of unsupervised children clambering on a jungle gym.

This book is an account of the emerging studies of human contact with the natural world and the resulting healing powers of nature, everything from trees, rocks, wind, sand, and even our relationship with formerly wild but now domesticated animals.

Evidence of this deep interrelationship with nature is well documented on the cave walls of the Périgord in France. Here and elsewhere around the world are the painted and scratched forms of our fellow travelers—wild horses, bison, antelope, lions, bears, and woolly mammoths. The exact purpose of these well-drafted images is not clear, but there can be no doubt that the artists who painted them were skilled observers of nature.

These earliest works of art, whose vitality and fluid energy would not be depicted again until the Renaissance, according to art historians, may have been somehow connected with magical thinking, or religion, or they may have just been paintings, art for art's sake so to speak. Either way, as Ron McAdow's essay, "The Enduring Animal," makes clear, human-animal mutualism eventually resulted in the domestication of certain species of wild animals. And perhaps not surprisingly, it turns out that association with animals is good for our health.

Further evidence of the deep connection with nature and human health can be found in the ancient knowledge of plants and their uses among people of what are currently termed preliterate cultures, the so-called medicine men, shamans, and curanderos. The traditions of these tribal groups goes back millennia, well before recorded time, and some of the cures they used, the surviving ones at least, must have had beneficial effects. In fact, as Teri Dunn Chace points out in her story, "The Garden of Earthly Cures," scientists from the industrialized world are well aware of this and have sent out botanical researchers to the uttermost ends of the earth in search of new cures from ancient medicines.

Perhaps even more significant, as far as the human species is concerned, is the fact that the young world in which we children of an industrial and agricultural society came of age was a green and florid landscape consisting of glades, marshes, wide savannahs, hills and mountains, green valleys and forests. Even today, mere visual exposure to this verdant world seems to have a calming and salutary effect, lowering blood pressure, slowing the heart rate, and even releasing a flood of hormones that induce a sense of well-being.

Illustrations of the ancient intimacy between people and nature are well known. The first cave paintings of animals were discovered in Spain and France in the nineteenth century and have been a subject of study ever since. And in the New World, the hunt for medicinal plants reaches back to the eighteenth century, and fostered some major scientific findings, including, incidentally, Darwin's discovery of evolution. Furthermore, for years now, anecdotally, contact with nature has been believed to impart beneficial health effects. But what is just now emerging is the scientific research and subsequent documentation of the physiological mechanisms of the beneficial effects of nature in healing and in the maintenance of mental and physical health.

The essays in this book document the various aspects of these new discoveries, including the combined mental and physical benefits of exposure to green space, even in small green urban parks; or association with natural objects and animals carried into institutions where people are confined indoors. Some of these stories, such as Thomas Conuel's "The Heart of the Matter" and Karl Meyer's "Places Between Bus Stops" are personal accounts of the mental and physical sanctuary that nature can offer.

Other stories document the unexpected health benefits to our brain chemistry as a result of time spent outdoors, and a few are excerpts from earlier works on the subject such as Edward O. Wilson's theory of biophilia and Richard Mabey's account of lifting his depression through his observations of swifts. Also included in this book, and tying the various essays together, is what is an elemental expression of the human reaction to contact with nature—poetry.

There are, however, currently two major threats to our ability to come together with the ancient rhythms of nature. In order to attain the health benefits from nature, we have to, as Thoreau pointed out, make contact with nature. And in a world where adults and, nowadays children as well, are cut off from the natural world by an addictive attachment to electronic devices, that contact is hard to achieve. We may learn facts about nature from computers and television programs, but encounter no real immersion in the wild world, no rich scent from the morning forest, no birdsong, no fragrance of flowers, nor feel of the moist skin of frogs, or of the rough underside of cleavers or lady's thumb. This aspect of the break with nature and what we can do to restore it is documented by Michael J. Caduto's story, "Children of the Wired World."

Finally, in order to have contact with nature, we must have wild nature, and as we know, worldwide, there is massive habitat destruction in progress, with over half of the world's wildlife populations gone in a matter of a few generations. Ann Prince's story, "Wildness and Wellness," addresses this loss, touches on the communion with nature that motivates land conservationists, and expands on the efforts of individuals and groups around the globe to preserve wildland for the sake of human health and happiness.

But the overarching point of this book, the singular commonality, is the basic fact that nature is good for us. It is preventative medicine, and it has a multiplicity of healing effects—yet one more good argument for preserving nature. Nature cures, and in order to maintain its benefits we have to save it—all of it—rocks, trees, wind, and water.

JHM, Editor

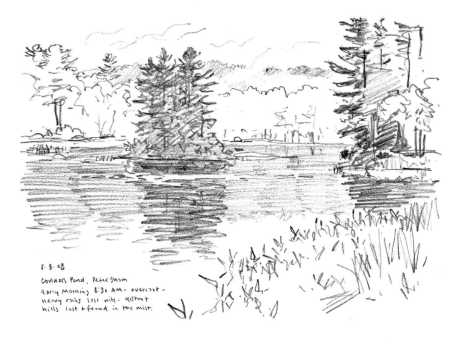

8.8.08
Connors Pond, Peterborough
Early morning 6:30 AM - overcast -
heavy rains last nite - distant
hills lost + found in the mist.

Lake

by Holly Guran

come toward me
bring me your waters

leave me to the loons
who call out in the night
for one another

needing only
an occasional breath,
coo-cakoo, a little hitch, an echo

waters come toward me
when I enter
loosen all of me

let the years that cling
on land swim to the far shore—

The Right Place
by Edward O. Wilson

First, the savanna itself, with nothing more added, offered an abundance of animal and plant food to which the omnivorous hominids were well adapted, as well as the clear view needed to detect animals and rival bands at long distances. Second, some topographic relief was desirable. Cliffs, hillocks, and ridges were the vantage points from which to make a still more distant surveillance, while their overhangs and caves served as natural shelters at night. During longer marches, the scattered clumps of trees provided auxiliary retreats sheltering bodies of drinking water. Finally, lakes and rivers offered fish, mollusks, and new kinds of edible plants. Because few natural enemies of man can cross deep water, the shorelines became natural perimeters of defense.

Put these three elements together: it seems that whenever people are given a free choice, they move to open tree-studded land on prominences overlooking water. This worldwide tendency is no longer dictated by the hard necessities of hunter-gatherer life. It has become largely aesthetic, a spur to art and landscaping. Those who exercise the greatest degree of free choice, the rich and powerful, congregate on high land above lakes and rivers and along ocean bluffs. On such sites they build palaces, villas, temples, and corporate retreats. Psychologists have noticed that people entering unfamiliar places tend to move toward towers and other large objects breaking the skyline. Given leisure time, they stroll along shores and riverbanks. They look along the water and up, to the hills beyond or to high buildings, expecting to see the sacred and beautiful places, the sites of historic events, now the seats of government, museums, or the homes of important personages. And they often do, in such landmarks as the Zähringen-Kyburg fortress of Thun, the Belvedere palace of Vienna, the cathedral in Saint Étienne, the Chateau of Angers, and the Potala, and among the more imposing sites from past eras,

Thingvellir, location of the ancient parliament of Iceland, the Parthenon, and the great plaza at Tenochtitlán.

The most revealing manifestation of triple criterion occurs in the principle of landscape design. When people are confined to crowded cities or featureless land, they go to considerable lengths to recreate an intermediate terrain, something that can tentatively be called the savanna gestalt. At Pompeii the Romans built gardens next to almost every inn, restaurant, and private residence, most possessing the same basic elements: artfully spaced trees and shrubs, beds of herbs and flowers, pools and fountains, and domestic statuary. When the courtyards were too small to hold much of a garden, their owners painted attractive pictures and plants and animals on the enclosure walls—in open geometric assemblages. Japanese gardens, dating from the Heian period of the ninth to twelfth centuries (and hence ultimately Chinese in origin), similarly emphasize the orderly arrangement of trees and shrubs, open space, and streams and ponds. The trees have been continuously bred and pruned to resemble those of the tropical savanna in height and crown shape. The

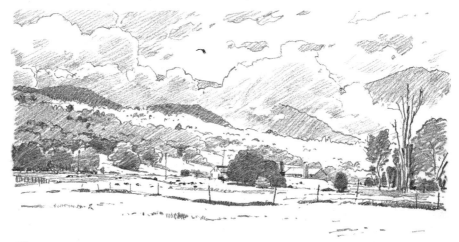

Stowe Vermont - View toward Mt Mansfield
July 11, 1992

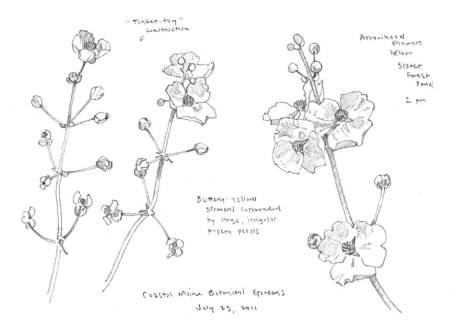

"Tinker-toy" construction

Arrowhead Flowers below
Slater Forest Pond
2 pm

Buttery-yellow stamens surrounded by large, irregular papery petals

Coastal Maine Botanical Gardens
July 25, 2011

dimensions are so close as to make it seem that some unconscious force has been at work to turn Asiatic pines and other northern species into African acacias.

I will grant at once the strangeness of the comparison and the possibility that the convergence is merely a large coincidence. It is also true the individuals often yearn to retain the dominant and sometimes peculiar qualities of the environment in which they were raised. But entertain for a while longer the idea that the landscape architects and gardeners, and we who enjoy their creations without special instruction or persuasion, are responding to a deep genetic memory of mankind's optimal environment. That given a completely free choice, people gravitate statistically toward a savanna-like environment. The theory accommodates a great many seemingly disconnected facts from other parts of the world. ❧

Biophilla by Edward O. Wilson, copyright © 1984 by the President and Fellows of Harvard College.

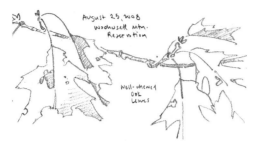

August 25, 2008
Woonsocket Mtn.
Reservation

Well-chewed
Oak
Leaves

I come out early

by Kathy Nelson

the sun one thumb's length
above the farthest trees,
to walk the morning road, the soft dirt tracked
by heavy tires, shaded by the fringed mimosas,
maples, poplars, others
whose names have slipped away,

and sunlit stones have long shadows,
and Queen Anne's lace leans along the fence,
and a robin drops down,
sudden raptor to a rattling June bug,
and in the field hay bales bask beside
the baler, quiet now, and in another,

six black cows dip their heavy heads
into deep grass, chewing, lashing their tails,
and from the house next to the field a rooster
calls out clear and high, and trellised vines
climb like lines of new recruits over the hill.
I've come out to find my bearings.

Let me say it another way: I am
the child of ones who walked a road like this,
and even though their road was dust

and their trees were scrub cedars,
their flowers thistles, nettles,
cattails on the river, and hawks ravaged

hapless squirrels, and red cows scrabbled
among burr-grass, and even though
they walked along their road to harvest
cotton fields that promised bleeding hands
and aching backs, still it is their road
I walk, looking for landmarks, signposts.

Birds singing

by Jack Kerouac

Birds singing
in the dark
—Rainy dawn.

One flower

by Jack Kerouac

One flower
on the cliffside
Nodding at the canyon

Places Between Bus Stops
The Restorative Power of Unlikely Walks
by Karl Meyer

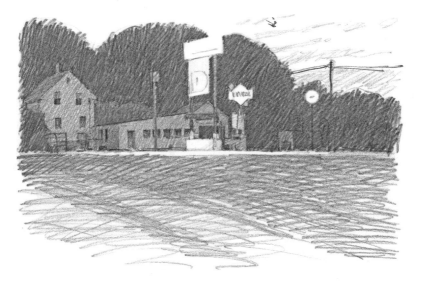

"I like walking because it is slow, and I suspect that the mind, like the feet, works at about three miles an hour. If this is so, then modern life is moving faster than the speed of thought, or thoughtfulness." Rebecca Solnit

Countless studies tout the benefits of walking: balance, creativity, emotional stability, physical health. Walking also offers revelation, the possibility of discovering new places. But it is the fact that my footsteps touch upon the stories of others and ground me on the planet that matters most. I get to see and listen in earth time. And the best days can be charmingly, exotically freeing for a quiet plodder such as myself, sniffing around old towns and rarely trammeled places. Padding along in a minimal carbon footprint, I find that past and present sometimes merge in moments that are downright exquisite.

I was deep in thought on a recent walk when an SUV pulled up and the driver leaned out and asked if I would like a ride. This was Herb who'd repaired my computer a few times when I lived up this way. I'd just crossed into Shelburne Falls on a walk along the Deerfield from East Charlemont through parts of Buckland. "No thanks," I said, "but thanks for asking."

"But you're limping," he noted, a bit concerned.

"Actually," I said, "I've been limping since I was twenty. If I stop limping, I'll stop limping."

There's some truth to that last statement. My right hip is an inch higher than the left one—not by design. Some people notice the hitch in my gate, but most don't. Still, I'm always grateful to be moving about the landscape under my own power. But I almost blew all that once—in one of those course-altering moments that occur in life. Though some take time and reflection to recognize, this one was different.

This one transpired under a blistering August sun on the desert prairie of north Texas. For several minutes, broken and bleeding, I wasn't sure I'd walk again. I'd just failed to vault over a looming guardrail from the back of a speeding motorcycle— my ragged skeleton cartwheeling several times before coming to a halt. And there I lay like crumpled paper; an unspeakable pain hammered my extremities.

Someone finally came to help me out of a fogging helmet. An ambulance had been summoned. "Hang on, I'll be back," he said, running off to locate the motorbike's injured driver. It was then that I finally looked down at ripped jeans and some oddly turned legs that didn't seem to be my own. I turned away, wanting to disappear into the Texas hardpan. But beyond that pain, there was also a profound numbness separating me from those odd-angled legs. They no longer felt part of me. Under assault, my mind and body seemed to have parted ways.

At 50 miles an hour I'd made hash of all the strongest bones in the body. I knew then something more was required. I was 20 years old and had to know: "Will I walk again?" Summoning all my courage I turned to face the moment. Against electrifying pain—and observing from what seemed a great distance, I gasped as my right knee twitched; then nudged up half an inch. "I'll live," I told myself, crumbling back in shock. That dodgy self-assessment likely helped save me.

Two months and five days later I left Wichita Falls General Hospital, rail thin and barely able to take a few steps. I wasn't well enough to travel home, but I was in love. I'd continue recuperating at the apartment of one of the nurse's aides who'd held my hand through weeks of surgeries and traction. It was absurdly romantic. My angel's name was Karen.

Yet amongst those weeks of developing romance were endless days when no one visited. I'd only been in Texas for weeks before the crash—my people were all in New Jersey. Healing time crept by slowly; sometimes not at all. August drifted to September, which lumbered on into October. Dead center in Tornado Alley, fall settled in heavy and still, its light strange. Billowing storms flashed past hospital windows, yet I couldn't detect any change in the season.

I daydreamed of home—of friends, familiar sights. But it was more than just a longing for things known. I craved my little corner of earth. My most fervent desire—one still tangibly sharp today, was to simply shuffle, ankle deep, through a pile of October leaves.

It's been two years since Herb pulled up and offered me that lift. I live in Greenfield and close to town these days—where I often leave my car idle in the driveway for a week or more. I walk almost daily, more purposely in winter for the sun and its helpful shot of vitamin D. In warmer months I move alternately by foot and bicycle, sometimes both. No matter the means, that quiet travel fulfills a longing to understand landscape and habitat, and to tread lightly across fertile tracts.

And I always go untethered, without a cell phone or iPod. People today seem indifferent to their surroundings in proportion to the amount of digital armor weighing them down. Out in the world, they're literally elsewhere—peering at screens telling them when to step left or right. We blithely wrap ourselves in the ever-spreading electric grid that's now overheating our habitat—while denying any interdependence on what's literally under our feet. We've allowed ourselves to become a pod race of savants, vulnerable to interruptions of electromagnetic pulses that can instantly pitch our daily lives all into an apoplectic stupor.

I was a full year recovering from that motorbike accident—three aspirin at a time, four times a day. Left with a tilted axis, I understood the need to keep moving—in order to keep moving. But somehow when I was able, it really wasn't a burden.

Before Texas, I'd barely been out of New Jersey. Most of my recovery year was ultimately spent there. Immobile and youthfully poor, I started reading: Melville, Dickens, Emerson, Conrad, Kerouac, Dostoyevsky, Faulkner, and, thankfully, Thoreau. My world got a little bigger. When I was at last well enough to support myself, my first purchases were hiking shoes and a bicycle. They'd keep me moving.

That day along the Deerfield I was actually working, being paid something as I walked. These last six years I've supported a modest lifestyle by driving a bus—which might seem anomalous to someone who prefers to turn his back on his carbon-belching car and hasn't boarded a plane in two decades. Suffice to say, it's what's working for me at the moment.

I mainly drive high schoolers to sporting events, museums, amusement parks, and science fairs. Though there's little glamour, it is mass transportation—efficient from an environmental standpoint. And though I was once a very disagreeable teen, today I'm pretty sympathetic, and happy to be working around their youthful energy. Am I highly paid? No. Are there big benefits? Not so much. But—in one way…yes.

In between transport, there is downtime. I can linger to watch the kids play—or root around the museum they're visiting. Or better yet, I can get my feet moving and poke around the setting onto which we've just descended. Many of my trips are nearby, but some can be two hours distant—from Massachusetts into Connecticut, Vermont, or New Hampshire. To me, walking is my own benefit. I'm paid something for my time, but it's up to me to enrich that compensation.

So I go exploring, which often informs my writing. And, in doing so, I realize that I'm always treading ancient paths—walking atop other people's stories. Present and past do literally merge when you wander into a seventeenth-century graveyard huddled in the shadows of Hartford's downtown towers. I go searching for the seeds of place. Who was here first? When? Why on this bend of river?

On longer trips I might cover 5 or 6 miles tromping a landscape or exploring a riverside—or haunting the frayed edges of eighteenth-century New England towns.

My walks bend quickly toward the past—seeking out the oldest house, the earliest gravestone, an old ferry landing—or a town's first mill site near an old stone bridge. On rural trips it might be ancient woods or a river crossing bearing an Algonquian name. Faced with the frenzied pace of our techno-consumer society, I'm hunting a language of place. It's my attempt to recover some essence of earth.

I've always had an inescapable awareness that history is much more than the acceptance of dry scholarly tales. I don't enter a city or town center without thinking—or knowing—that this place was once home to others: Deerfield was once Pocumtuck and Springfield was once Agawam. It never slips my mind that there is a Hockanum in Hadley and another south of the state border in East Hartford—both sites cradled in the shadow of an ancient Connecticut River oxbow. And it never leaves me that the people who first adopted those names for places they knew as home did so in a deliberate tongue that connected them to what they understood as the essence of their earth.

Everywhere we tread, no matter how indecipherable a modern landscape has become, it once had another name and another language—relayed in sounds that strove to offer its history and significance to its denizens. Those names were a key to an unbroken human connection to earth. Nearly all of that was erased. We are often left with just fragments.

That's why I was once dumbstruck to discover that a young Protestant immigrant and colonial trader named Roger Williams took time in 1643 to write *A Key into the Language of America*, translating Algonquian phrases for the English tongue. That opened a door for me, just a crack. A white spire may still be a great comfort to a little Massachusetts town, but just three centuries back the raising of that steeple signaled subjugation and conquest to still-living peoples whose ancestors had walked here for thousands of years prior.

"I believe in the forest, and in the meadow, and in the corn that grows in the night," Thoreau wrote in his essay "Walking"—a swipe at rote Yankee preaching that exhorted ultimate dominance of the lands and landscapes so recently annexed. Today we rush across places where seminal cultures were brutally shattered and dispersed—conquests that, in very short order, led to the wholesale devouring of age-old New England forests.

So I go in search of a language of land. That may seem quaint in a time when Downtown Crossing is most identified as a collecting point for Boston consumers. Or here, Hadley—a 1659 Connecticut River settlement identified as Norwottuck on early maps—is now most notable for its ever-expanding mall strip near Old Bay Road. That's part of what motivates me to walk. And I also think that maybe the earth talks to us a little bit through our feet, reveals some of its stories. We just seem to have stopped listening—perhaps when we abandoned walking to race across the earth in the hardened shells of carbon-spewing conveyances.

There's a leafy amusement park in North Granby, Connecticut—relatively pleasant and not overly electrified. One could be tempted to just sit by the shaded pool there. Instead I headed out in mid-June heat along a narrow stretch of Route 189. After a mile I veered off at Day Street—an intersection flanked by an old farmhouse. That led me up along the ridge overlooking the Salmon Brook Valley. Most of the houses turned out to be newer, with little pasture remaining. But then came a break in that developed tract—an opening where the light appeared different.

What popped out next—monstrously sprawling and stubbornly clinging to life was the Dewey-Granby Oak. It was simply stunning, and all the more so set along this old road—holding ground against a spreading suburban shadow. I recognized its name from some distant reading, but knew nothing more. Here, unannounced and magnificent, was that sun-dappled great oak—a specimen worthy of period films set on old English estates.

But truth be told, there was little in the way of detail to adhere to. Rooted here long ago, the Dewey-Granby Oak simply remains a presence to this day. Someone must've taken a core sample when this patch of earth was preserved by the Granby

Land Trust. A plaque from 1997 intoned it had begun life perhaps 450 years earlier. However accurate, that implied that it was just a forest ridge seedling at the time of Shakespeare's birth in 1564. The native Tunxis people who were then traveling this trail, which later became Day Street, passed and repassed a white oak growing to maturity. Yet little more than a century on, Europeans began swarming into this little valley, quickly felling the upland tracts to stump pastures. An ancient woodland path disappeared beneath cart ruts and grazing cattle, with only one venerable wolf tree left as witness.

Here then was my day's clue to understanding a moment in time. Survival, longevity, green leaves sprouted along sprawling weathered branches. I'm not sure exactly why that satisfied me. Yet unheralded bits of knowledge are often what offer context to the fabric of life. I paused there for a few minutes, breathing in the continuity of a long life. "I have great faith in a seed," Thoreau wrote. Today my seed was an old oak.

Wilder hikes on bus trips are rare, but there was a recent scramble up Mount Monadnock. We hustled up; then down, to deliver the dozens of prep schoolers we'd unleashed on that hill. But briefly, in between, there were grand three-state views connecting back to another companion who'd passed this way. Thoreau visited here a handful of times, finding Monadnock a worthy place to "go a-fishin'."

Thoreau and I would meet again on a trip to Bellows Falls High. A walk there brought me to the train stop near the Connecticut River where Thoreau once disembarked. Unbeknownst to me, he'd also once walked to the Great Eddy—an ancient Abenaki fishing site below the falls. Into the late 1700s, Yankee farmers could still pull up 1,200 American shad here in a single haul of the net.

But Thoreau and I were both disappointed by the Connecticut River. For Thoreau it was that there was hardly any river at all, the lingering result of the navigation canal diversion for riverboats, just upstream. Mine is the fact that those migrating shad—a half-century after Congress authorized the four-state Connecticut River migratory fisheries restoration, still fail to reach Bellows Falls.

From day one, shad were the program's key restoration species. Far from extinct today, most remain blocked and imperiled 50 miles downstream—trapped in the private power canal below Turners Falls Dam at the place once called Peskeomskut. Though a small portion of the run squeezes upstream toward open Massachusetts, Vermont, and New Hampshire habitats—some 200,000 shad or more never make it past a dam where they've been blocked since 1798.

Winter 2015 wasn't easy for ambulation. Still, a mid-February trip to Phillips Exeter Academy in New Hampshire had its highlights. Though sidewalks were lined in waist-deep snow, I tramped Exeter's centuries-old byways for hours. I bundled down to the Squamscott River and its old bridge and frozen fishway. A turkey vulture swooped in—yards above the snowy street, the surprise of a brief squall. Sculptor Daniel Chester French's birthplace is marked in downtown Exeter—along with the first meeting site of the Republican Party. Historic houses are now festooned with the symbol of an alewife, or smelt—ancient staples of the Pennacook and those who came after.

But my best walk came in mid-April, though dingy snow piles still had plenty of life in them. I'd dropped my kids off at Lowell National Historic Park. The forecast wasn't great—brooding, with showers expected, but the temperature was nearing sixty. I had hours to burn, and a rain jacket, so I took to the streets. I'd been here once, briefly in midwinter. The Merrimack, Pawtucket Falls, and Lowell's ragged bordering neighborhoods grabbed my fancy. I'd wanted more.

This April day, winter seemed finally ready to relent. The rain held off as I steered toward Market Street, where the Olympic Bakery had offered me a great Greek salad and fresh cannoli last time. The sun burst through in a neighborhood of unvarnished factory houses. I ordered pizza slices to go and found a quiet doorway where I sat in the late morning's humid air. Then I headed to the river.

I was dreaming of the Merrimack's shad runs of old—wondering if endangered shortnose sturgeon had ever spawned this high in its reaches. Landlords were chipping away at stubborn ice, and the gates leading to the Riverwalk remained closed, still snowed over. But I followed the Merrimack just the same, heading downstream on Pawtucket Street and crossing at the first opportunity. This landed me at the edge of UMass Lowell's North Campus overlooking the city's old mill towers. Ruminating on that bank, I reflected that the earth under me was once part and parcel of a Pennacook village here.

The showers remained at bay so I continued seaward beside the water—crossing the river four times at 3 historic bridge sites. I gained a new sense of Lowell's Byzantine canal system—branching from, and linking, the Concord and Merrimack. As hydraulics got refined, the rivers and river travel here were quickly eclipsed by giant mills and locomotives. Farther on, I stumbled into a tiny urban park honoring Jack Kerouac. Enshrined on a polished slab was one of his poems, a loving edgy retelling of his parents' stark lives here and his own subsequent birth along hard-bit Merrimack shores. It lent a presence to the place.

My best minutes came farther along, at the merging place of two branching canals not far from Lowell's rust-brick downtown and signature Lowell Sun Building. I'd walked back in time along remnants of the centuries-old navigation system to its convergence with the Concord River, just ahead. Here, some 175 years prior, young Henry Thoreau and his brother, John, had passed—heading through locks ushering them onto the Merrimack. They steered upriver on that larger stream—north toward New Hampshire towns that were already felling their last forests to fuel an Industrial Revolution. Under that warming April sun, my day's walk somehow seemed complete.

But there's another walking exploration I've repeatedly engaged in these last four years—my tornado walk. I've literally been walking around inside a tornado. On June 1, 2011, an astonishing EF3 tornado touched down in West Springfield. It skipped across the Connecticut; then battered the landscape for a full 39 miles east—all the way to Southbridge. I'd been driving kids through West Springfield just the day before it thundered through.

Tornadoes stalked the dreams of my youth since childhood, likely an offshoot of viewing *The Wizard of Oz*. Though these violent storms are strangely fascinating, I've never hankered to experience one in the flesh. In dreams they'd always loomed ominously on the periphery—never quite catching me up. But the absolute destructive power of this one—here in the Northeast—was disturbingly eye-opening. Three people died; hundreds of homes were destroyed. It roared across towns in a traceable half-mile-wide trajectory, just south of Route 20—in places where my bus trips often intersect.

That fall at West Springfield's Eastern States Expo, I walked out the gate and into the neighborhoods due north. Whole houses still lay in ruins, dozens uninhabitable. Thousands of windows had imploded and were boarded up, or were being replaced. What trees remained were hulks, stripped of all lateral branches. At Union Street the devastation across tightly clustered double- and triple-decker apartment homes was withering. A mother died here while shielding her teenage daughter from the storm's fury. Heading home on I-91, Springfield's South End was yet a mass of tumble-brick ruins. In the distance, a checkerboard of tarped roofs led up the ridge toward East Forest Park like it was a staircase painted in blue.

One snowy day the following December, I again walked that tornado's course among the relict trees south of Wilbraham Center. Cars had skittered off the highway, but I got my kids settled in safe. I then bundled up and took off down Main Street, where that unseen power had descended with little warning six months prior. It peeled off roofs, toppled outbuildings, and shattered scores of trees—then stalked off up the mountain ridge toward Monson. One displaced citizen had returned to string up holiday lights on her darkened uninhabitable home.

In late February I took another walk in that great scar where—just minutes later that June day, the tornado barreled down the ridge into Monson Center. Snap, snap—snap, snap, snap!—like twigs, whole trees were crowned; stems jackknifed just 20 feet from the ground. The storm roared off to the east.

And I did the same, later that spring—on a Sturbridge Village trip. It's just a ten-minute walk out the back of that museum to where that EF3 twister roared in, devouring an entire wooded swamp. It snapped and scattered trunks in astonishing blow-down jumbles, then crossed Route 131 into Southbridge.

On a return trip to Wilbraham two Aprils ago, I backtracked into that storm's path once more. After dropping off my busload I followed a hunch into the landscape. Peepers and warblers called along a winding cross-country trail leading through lowland woods. But then a new slant of light from a little bluff to the north caught my eye. That detour—just a few yards off the trail—brought me dead center into the storm. Helter-skelter before me lay the remnants of a once-broad, upland forest—mature pine, oak and maple, leveled, upended; dead. Hundreds of trees, rank-on-rank—tossed or tumbled, sucked up; then mowed down, like bowling pins.

The devastation was stark and powerful, yet bits of the place were now returning to life. A few trees, pitched and leaning, struggled on. Flickers and nuthatches darted about the edges, feasting on the buggy decay. The trail wound back down, and widened to a swampy marsh, also raked by the storm. Here too were the crowned haphazardly blown trees of a wetland—shorn of branches and left as lifeless hulks. But in the crook of one was a fat jumble of sticks. And there, in profile, sat an erect great blue heron. I quickly counted four more nests and attending sentinels occupying four more of those hulks. Astonishing.

My storm walk in Wilbraham continued this last spring. In mid-April there was but one active heron nest remaining. Wood frogs had arisen from the ground just the day before, but they were quiet. The females had yet to join the gathering. Still I understood that this was a place becoming—a landscape evolving. And that's part of the reason I'll likely take this same walk again, if it happens to turn up on my assigned bus route.

Beyond these unlikely locations, though, there's one particular walk I'm absolutely certain I'll be taking. Every fall, randomly and unannounced, blue sky and a hint of early October chill takes hold of me. Then, for a brief few minutes, I'll joyously drag my clumsy feet through a pile of autumn leaves—relishing the decay they stir into the air and savoring a papery sound that says home.

Oxygen

by Susan Edwards Richmond

Eight egrets float on the marsh fringe,
one, two, three at a time, rising,
falling back into brushstrokes.

If I hadn't sat, I wouldn't have seen them,
or just now, the kingfisher, arrested in air,
heavy bill, slightly parted, pointing down

before the dive, the lilies overblown
into alien pods, the cattails turning
inside out their tufts of fur.

I am convinced more than ever
it is oxygen I need,
the unadulterated air.

But where? Last night we hurried in
at dusk to shut up the house
against the sprayers' poison.

Out here, I still feel the crackle
of an airway lapsed, the muscular
gymnastics of long-term Lyme.

But this morning creeps
across the rail in the yellow jacket's
bands, the swallowtail's buoyant

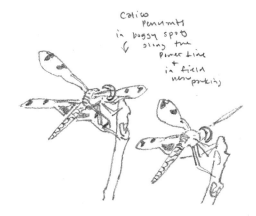

refusal to light. Marsh wind
blows my hair clean
over acres and acres—

it looks like you could walk
from here to those egrets.
But you can't.

They are comfortable in distance.
I want to tell you—
but the words haven't been invented yet.

Until you hear the buzzing
in your own head,
I tell you this instead.

The Natural Mind
In an Urbanized Digitalized World, We Need Nature More Than Ever
by Nini Bloch

According to a 2011 study of 30 years of data assessing empathy among American college students in North America over the last three decades, the ability to respond emotionally to someone else's distress, in other words display empathy, has declined almost 50 percent. This downward trend in empathy tracks a parallel 50 percent drop in nature-based recreation over the past 40 years.

Is this merely a coincidence or are these two statistics related in some deeper way?

Mounting scientific evidence suggests that indeed these statistics are intimately tied to each other, especially when one considers another statistic. Currently, 81 percent of Americans live in cities, and now—for the first time in history—so does half the rest of the world's population. As the US has become more urbanized and digitized, we have turned our backs on nature with disturbing consequences for individual health and society's well-being. Particularly worrying is the escalation of stress-based, chronic conditions and, with declining empathy, a decrease in the desire to help others and an increase in narcissism and self-absorption in young adults.

Neuroscientists are currently making significant strides in understanding how the human brain works and how our screen-driven, fast-paced urban lifestyle is challenging that mass of neurons inside our skulls that evolved to deal with a much different setting—the natural world. The result is that we are actually changing the configuration of our brains. Researchers have discovered that not only are we instinctively attracted to nature but that it has profound, positive effects on our moods, decisions, behavior—and health. Scientists have also learned that—as much as we pride ourselves on our highly evolved neocortex, the thinking part of the brain—it's actually the much older "emotional brain" that runs the show. Neurochemistry drives our feelings and shapes our health.

The veritable storm of insights that have resulted from this research offers both hope and a road map for restructuring our brains, improving our health, and reversing the trend away from nature. Already, individuals and even nations are applying the principles, encouraging activities such as taking a mindful walk in the woods—with proven results—happier less-stressed souls.

It has taken considerable effort to bring to light the scientific underpinnings of what we knew in the first place—watching a sunset is good for us. Countless poems and works of art have celebrated nature's deep effect on our souls, but until relatively recently scientists have largely skirted the subject. Delving into the possible health benefits that immersion in nature might confer on us received the scientific cold shoulder because any reputed results were based largely on self-reported emotions rather than hard data: "I feel better; I don't feel as stressed."

Scientists deemed emotions too immeasurable, "squishy," and complex to investigate. At best, psychology approached emotions sideways, isolating them from the brain's functions. Getting hard data about the brain's reactions to nature required, first, probing what part of the brain was triggered by exposure to nature, and, second, understanding what the brain was doing to the body. Only then could we understand the nature–brain link. The brain itself remained a black box; however, we couldn't peer inside it to see what was actually going on.

Now, with new tools like electroencephalograms (EEGs) and functional magnetic resonance imaging (fMRIs) and more advanced analyses of the suite of chemicals the brain produces, we are beginning to piece together how the 3-pound organ inside our skulls works. Both EEGs and fMRIs pinpoint where in the brain neurons are firing in response to a thought, feeling, or action. These tools are becoming portable, meaning that the scientists can take them into the field and get real-time data about the brain's reactions to life outside the lab.

Our brains are both complex, integrated electric switching stations (with trillions of pathways connecting roughly 100 billion neurons to each other) and sophisticated factories that produce cascades of powerful neurochemicals (such as cortisol, which signals stress). Brains are busy places; they have to be to keep the body's basic functions running smoothly yet take in and respond to all manner of stimuli, form memories, learn new things, and revise responses. Brains are never static. They're constantly in flux, adapting and forming new neuron networks as unused ones wither or are damaged (for instance, by a stroke). We call this neuroplasticity, and it's a hallmark of our species. The brain's capacity to alter its chemistry and its very structure can profoundly modify behavior for better or worse.

Much current research has focused on the emotional, or limbic, brain, which lies between the neocortex (the thinking logical part of the brain) and the brain stem (the oldest most primitive part of the brain that controls functions like heart rate, digestion, respiration, and balance). The emotional brain that we inherited from mammals generates many primal emotions (fear, anger, desire) and forms memories. The emotional brain belies our faith in ourselves as rational beings because it tends to shoot first and ask questions later.

In other words, it's often "blurted out" some chemical response to a situation before it confers with the neocortex. To a greater or lesser extent, we are ruled by our emotional brains, which evolved way before humans ever acquired language. Only now are we beginning to understand how the emotional brain shapes our feelings, decisions, behavior, and what we become. Poet and musician Sidney Lanier held that the initial step of every plan and every action is an emotion—a rather apt description of what really goes on in our brains.

To understand how nature affects our health, it helps to consider what our brains evolved to do. The human brain has had two million years to evolve, two centuries to contend with the Industrial Revolution, and perhaps three decades to cope with global urbanization and the Digital Age. In the beginning, early humans wandered in hunter-gatherer bands. They were highly mobile, had no set shelter, and figured out on the fly how to get fruit, hunt small animals, and avoid getting eaten. This description aligns nicely with molecular biologist John Medina's assertion that our brains evolved to "solve problems related to surviving in an unstable outdoor environment, and to do so in nearly constant motion."

As with many other animals, we're hardwired to scan the environment for dangers (predators, avalanches) and opportunities (food, shelter). The new brain-measuring gadgetry and human subjects' reactions are confirming what we already intuitively know: we instinctively like open vistas. From a survival point of view, we want to be able to see what's coming our way. Lake and ocean shores, riverbanks, bluffs, prairies, mountain ranges, and open forests are all scenes we find particularly attractive—more so than almost any human-built scene.

Water has a special hold on us, and not only because it's essential for our survival. Researchers at Plymouth University in the UK reported that when they asked 40 adults to rate their preferences for either natural or built scenes in 100 photos, participants generally rated the green space photos higher. But any photo that contained water—even in an urban setting—rated highest. A water fountain in a town square draws people like a magnet. In the same vein, just think how the words "ocean view" or "lakefront property" jack up the sales price of real estate.

In their book *Your Brain on Nature: The Science of Nature's Influence on Your Health, Happiness, and Vitality*, Eva Selhub, MD, and Alan Logan, ND, note that our brain seems to operate on a Goldilocks principle. In the UK study, "There was a consistent attraction to water up to a certain point—scenes containing between 33 and 66 percent were, as Goldilocks would say, just right. Too much or too little water detracted from preference scores." That makes sense: a violent stormy sea would be threatening so it wouldn't garner preference points. In like manner, dense, dark forests are scary (imagine the foreboding woodlands of *Grimm's Fairy Tales*). Our brains try to find a balance in nature between boring simplicity and threatening chaos.

Human brains excel at picking out animals in settings and are acutely sensitive to animal movement, far more so than noticing trucks or baby carriages. Even babies, for instance, are attentive to animals more than inert toys. Our ancestors needed to be able to spot and determine quickly if a movement in the bush was a predator, prey, or just a falling mango. We are a species finely attuned to movement, but the frenetic pace of video games that kids play for hours on end and the loud music and strobe lights in bars are a far cry from watching the gentle lap of waves on a shore. One has to wonder what constant exposure to all the incessant flashing visuals and noise do to the brain.

Another human survival strategy is to pay more attention to "bad stuff." As marine biologist Wallace J. Nichols says in his book, *Blue Mind: The Surprising Science That Shows How Being Near, In, On, or Under Water Can Make You Happier, Healthier, More Connected, and Better at What You Do*, "Our brains are wired to be Teflon for the positive and Velcro for the negative to ensure our survival; we notice and react more strongly to negative experiences than to positive ones because otherwise we'd lackadaisically stroll our way to extinction." Our minds rapidly evaluate stimuli for their threat value, label them with emotional content, and, when necessary, issue the alarm that triggers the body's automatic fight-or-flight response. Emotionally and physically, this is an expensive response, so, ideally, it happens rarely; but in modern society it can become a daily experience—with chronic insidious effects.

We all experience daily hassles: traffic congestion, computer malfunctions, quarrels with coworkers, impatient people. Estimates are that North American adults face an average of 50 such irritations and inconveniences per day. We can't make the distinction between happening upon a coiled rattlesnake and encountering a surly repairman. This sets in motion "a cascade of stress physiology," as Selhub and Logan term it, especially causing an influx of the stress hormone cortisol. Cortisol sticks in your system for a couple of hours. Every time you encounter a hassle, your body is bathed in cortisol, and that carries long-term health risks. Chronic stress leads to inflammation and oxidative stress that damages cells in almost every system in the body, compromises the immune system, and feeds anxiety and depression. All these outcomes shorten life expectancy.

In order to eat, our hunter-gatherer ancestors had to explore and search for food. The urge to explore is in our blood, and the brain rewards the quest as much as the discovery. The brain's reward system reinforces risk taking, novel experiences, and physical effort with dopamine, a neurotransmitter that controls the brain's reward and pleasure centers, as well as regulating movement and emotional responses, which is why we keep on searching. Washington State University neuroscientist Jaak Panksepp has named this drive the seeking circuit and has found that seeking is self-rewarding: the process is fun and exciting.

Beachcombing, soccer, shopping, and surfing the Internet are all forms of seeking that we find entertaining. They give us intermittent rewards at irregular intervals and the hope that on that next rack is that perfect little black dress. The seeking circuit doesn't just kick in when we're hungry; it also operates when we're relaxed and happy. Its purest form is play. Learning is a natural outcome of searching.

A necessary corollary to the urge to explore and learn is that humans are stimulation junkies. Our brains demand input. Put a volunteer in a floatation tank that deprives him of all stimuli except touch, and for the first 45 minutes the brain typically sifts through the day's detritus. After that, the test subject gets tense and bored and then disoriented and confused and can even become delusional and hallucinate. Our hunger for stimulation drives many of us to spend up to one-third of every 24 hours on screens. Each interruption may cost us ten minutes to refocus on the original task, but our thirst for information and digital connection keeps us coming back to our screens.

Our fear that we'll "miss something"—in part fueled by social pressure—also feeds our compulsion, for example, to check text messages. The instant entertainment available on a screen makes us an impatient nation—and reinforces another tendency of the human brain. Nichols points out, "The emotional brain is hardwired to overvalue instant gratification and undervalue future rewards." Picture the child who's tried to save his allowance for a video game but has spent it all on soda and pizza instead. Humans may be innately programmed to live in the present.

When we concentrate on a task like doing taxes that involves conscious thinking and making decisions, our brain is constantly screening out all the other irrelevant "noise" that would distract us from the work at hand so that we can focus. Environmental psychologists Stephen and Rachel Kaplan call this "directed attention." As anyone who's done taxes or some other tedious work can attest, it's mentally exhausting mainly because of the effort required to maintain your attention on Form 1040 while filtering out all the extraneous signals—the cat knocking pens off your desk, for example, or the sound of the garbage truck grabbing your bin—or, hardest of all, inhibiting your mind's tendency to wander during the drudgery.

After doing taxes, your brain needs to rest. What scientists are discovering is that the best antidote to mental exhaustion is for the brain to go into a default mode in a natural setting. It's a state of relaxed alertness that Nichols refers to as "the Blue Mind state of calm centeredness." If you're walking along a familiar beach, you may notice in passing the extra seaweed last night's storm cast up on the shore or a gull dining on a dead fish, but these events will only perk your interest for an instant. Your senses are engaged, you're very much in the present, but you're not actively focusing on anything. The Kaplans labeled this state "involuntary attention." Involuntary attention is easy; it doesn't seem to take much energy or effort.

"Scientists now theorize that the default-mode network allows the brain to consolidate experiences and thus prepare to react to environmental stimuli," says Nichols. This process requires copious "chatter" with the hippocampus, the brain center involved in creating new memories and learning. When your brain is in default mode, it's most likely to come up with novel solutions to problems and bursts of inspiration—"out of the blue"—because your brain is forming new connections. While the mind is busy consolidating, it allows your exhausted frontal lobes to rest and recharge. Brain centers linked to emotions, pleasure, and empathy take over at these times and measurably calm you, according to Nichols.

Unfortunately, this process doesn't work well in a human-built setting, and our mental, physical, and emotional health is suffering for it. With their noise, crowds, traffic, flashing neon lights, tight spaces, and beckoning stores, cities overwhelm us with distractions, clutter, and more stimuli—and choice— than our brains are naturally designed to cope with. We feel the strain of trying to both filter out the irrelevant signals and concentrate on what we need to. Prolonged periods of trying to fight off distractions to focus on a boring task can affect the brain's inhibition system, making us more prone to inappropriate outbursts. We kid ourselves that we're being doubly efficient by multitasking. There's little down time for the always-on lifestyle, so the brain can't shift into involuntary attention to recuperate, especially if there's no green space around.

Despite the brain's remarkable plasticity, the rush to urbanize and digitize our lives has outstripped its capacity to adapt to the artificial human-built landscape. The brain is an ancient organ coping as best it can to a new world. As a result, rates of stress, anxiety, and depression in the West are on the rise, as are prescriptions to treat them. On the positive side, there's more and more scientific evidence accumulating that immersion in nature is good for us, and programs applying the theory are taking hold. Tapping into the instinctive attraction humans feel toward nature and finding innovative ways to provide access to natural settings, especially in cities, is key to reversing the trend.

The Japanese have put a new spin on the oft-touted "morning constitutional." The Forest Agency of Japan pioneered the effort in 1982 by launching the

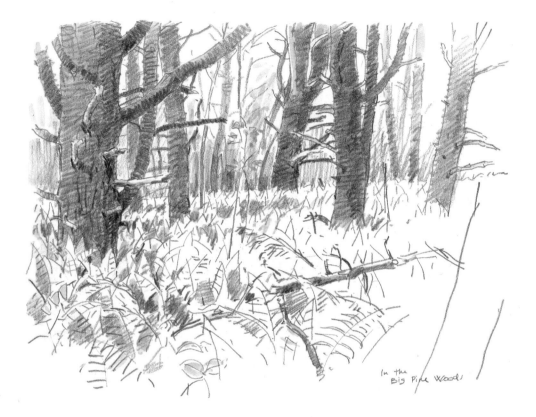

"In the Big Pine Woods"

shinrin-yoku (forest bathing) program. In practicing *shinrin-yoku*, the main idea is to experience the forest with all five senses rather than to get somewhere. This is by no means a power walk but a way to harmonize stressed physiology with the natural world, wordlessly. Anecdotally, forest bathing makes people happier: they approach the day's challenges with more of a spring in their step; they feel less stressed.

But could scientists prove the benefits?

Since forests cloak 64 percent of Japan, Forest Agency personnel had many sites to choose from and conducted a variety of experiments to test the value of forest bathing. In 1982 Yoshifumi Miyazaki, PhD, of Chiba University measured stress levels in subjects who had walked for 40 minutes either in some of the nation's oldest forests in Yakushima or in a laboratory setting. Not only did the forest walkers report better moods and being more invigorated, but their levels of cortisol were lower than for those who walked in the lab. Subsequent studies in other Japanese forests showed that *shinrin-yoku* also reduced blood pressure and pulse rate and increased heart rate variability (a measure of how well your circulatory system can cope with stress) when compared with walking in urban settings. The forest walkers slept better and reported fewer depressive symptoms and feelings of hostility than their city counterparts.

Researchers from Chiba University measured lower levels of oxygen in the prefrontal cortex of subjects walking in the forest. Since threats and hard mental or physical labor drive up levels of oxygen in this part of the brain, the result indicates that, as Selhub and Logan write, "The brain is taking a time-out while in the forest."

Indications that the brain is relaxing during *shinrin-yoku* led to another discovery: that reducing stress boosts the immune system in measureable ways. Qing Li, MD, of the Nippon Medical School documented increases in the number and the efficiency of natural killer cells (that attack viruses) and anticancer proteins after subjects walked as little as two hours in a forest. What's more, the boosted immunity lasted for a week or more after the walk(s). For middle-aged employees, two 1.5-mile forest walks per day over a weekend boosted their natural killer cell activity by 56 percent, and their immune function maintained a 23 percent increase for a full month. It seems clear that *shinrin-yoku* is good preventative medicine.

Researchers wondered, if two 1.5-mile walks in a Japanese forest over a weekend can boost your immune system for a whole month, what would a bigger dose of forest medicine do? With medical doctors, Won Sop Shin, PhD, conducted a nine-day camping trip (with activities like rock climbing) for college students suffering from depression. Although it's difficult to control for all the variables in such a venture, the students' post-trip depression scores dropped 64 percent—far better than the results of successful drug trials.

Part of the success of the nine-day camping trip may have been due to its more aerobic nature. We know that aerobic exercise by itself improves cognition, executive function, cell health, and blood flow to the brain. It aids the production of serotonin and chemicals that protect the brain. Exercise is a natural antidepressant that helps buffer stress, which improves mood. Studies have shown that exercise in a green space outperforms exercise in a gym. Outdoor activity increases a positive outlook and self-esteem, which makes it more likely that the exerciser will continue the program. Since our evolutionary heritage dictates that we were meant to be active, outdoor animals, these findings should come as no surprise.

Researchers found that other major contributors to boosting immunity during *shinrin-yoku* walks are the chemicals that trees, especially evergreens, release into the air to protect themselves from bacteria, fungi, and insects and that we breathe in. That familiar pine smell is one example. It seems odd that these so-called phytoncides should work so well both in humans and in trees, but Li has correlated the level of phytoncides in the air with increased immune-system performance. And phytoncides offer the gamut of sedative and energizing effects while reducing stress-hormone production and anxiety.

There is another unseen component of the atmosphere that benefits a forest walker: negative ions. In abundance in forests and near water around sunrise and sunset and after rainfall, negative ions enhance the human antioxidant defense system and blood flow. Subjects report that exposure to negative ions alleviates anxiety, depression, and stress, boosting cognitive performance. In contrast, enclosed spaces, air-conditioning, and electronic devices all tend to suck negative ions out of the atmosphere.

Researchers have found that other natural settings offer many of the same benefits. *Your Brain on Nature* makes the case on a communal, regional, or even national scale that just living close to natural areas may reduce the risk of disease and even mortality. In Japan, researchers noted that higher amounts of forest cover per prefecture protected inhabitants against six common cancers, and in Glasgow and Shanghai similar studies of land use data showed that areas with more green space correlated with lower risk of mortality. What was particularly remarkable, Selhub and Logan point out, is that green space appeared to be "a great equalizer": it wiped out much of the large disparity in health risks faced by the haves and the have-nots. This finding is a powerful endorsement for creating more urban parks.

The largest chunk of nature on the planet, of course, is the ocean. "Some 99 percent of our biosphere is water," says Nichols. He is a passionate conservationist who believes that you save what you love, and he loves water above all. His life is about turning his affection for water into the Blue Mind movement, as he calls it, starting with getting people in, on, under, and around our liquid world.

Nichols wants to kindle a love of oceans, lakes, and rivers in humanity to save both the planet and ourselves. To make his case, he began searching for a book detailing our emotional connection to water. There wasn't one, so he wrote it (*Blue Mind*). It turns out that the health benefits of experiences with bodies of water parallel those of forest medicine—with some notable differences.

We can immerse ourselves in water in a way we can't in air, and we've been doing so for centuries. Hot spring spas, whirlpools, cool showers, and swimming in the ocean all improve our psychological and physical well-being. Researchers have measured and documented that such activities lower cortisol, mental fatigue, anxiety, and muscular tension. With 600 times the resistance of air, water buoys and holds us.

Beyond the effects of actually being in water, the sound and sight are moving to us in surprising ways. Both marketing and scientific research confirm that blue is most people's favorite color, associated, Nichols says, with "trust, confidence, and dependable strength." You don't have to look far in the corporate world to find blue logos. Neurosurgeon Amir Vokshoor, MD, claims that the brain's response to the color blue mimics the effects of dopamine:

"feelings of euphoria, joy, reward, and wellness." There's evidence that watching a blue light enhances our ability to understand voices and increases sensitivity in the brain's centers for attention and memory. These are features that could ease communication.

One of the most mesmerizing qualities of any large body of water is the dance of light on its surface. Nichols surmises it was "the shiniest thing our ancestors saw." Equally transfixing is the irregular and unpredictable but familiar movement of waves. Our brains need such "creative disequilibrium," says Nichols, to recover from the onslaught of daily urban stimuli, from the monotonous hum of the refrigerator to the flickering lights and staccato sounds of fast-paced video games. We're drawn to the "combination of novelty and repetition," says Nichols. For that reason, we love to watch waves crashing on the beach, fountains, waterfalls, fires, shifting desert sands, billowing clouds, and prairie grasses blowing in the wind. We find it restful. We've shifted into Blue Mind mode.

One of the most oft-cited and convincing studies about nature's effect on physiology is Roger S. Ulrich's 1984 journal article in *Science* analyzing 10 years of records from a Pennsylvania hospital. It details the recovery of patients whose gallbladders had been removed, with the only variable being whether the recovery room looked out on a little forest or on a brick wall. Patients who enjoyed the forest view recovered faster with fewer postsurgical complications, used less potent pain medications, and earned fewer negative comments from the nurses than their brick-wall counterparts. Windows are good for our health, and hospitals and schools in particular are building accordingly. For windowless rooms, however, the best option may be bringing the outside in.

Researchers have wondered whether having a bit of nature inside offices, hospital rooms, and schools can help protect office workers, patients, and schoolchildren from the ravages of oxidative stress and the other doldrums of their digitized lives. The short answer is, yes, potted plants and aquariums do help. Adding one or several potted plants to a work space increased productivity, reaction time, memory recall, and ability to perform proofreading tasks—and elevated workers' moods and level of comfort as well. In Australia, middle school students' scores in math, science, and spelling increased 12 percent in classrooms six weeks after plants were brought in. Appendectomy patients recovering in a room with potted plants used fewer pain medications, had lower blood pressure and heart rate, and reported less anxiety, more energy, and more positive thoughts than similar patients in rooms without plants. A few potted plants in a room do seem to make people happier, reduce their stress, and enhance their cognitive functioning.

Dentists have aquariums in their waiting rooms because watching fish is proven to relax patients and lower blood pressure and heart rate, producing calmer, less anxious occupants in the dentist's chair. The more species of fish in the tank, the more the heart rate drops. We can assume that working for extended periods in rooms with plants improves worker health overall. In one study plants in a hospital setting reduced employees' short-term sick leave by 60 percent. That saves hospitals money.

Spending time in nature seems critical to triggering empathy and an altruistic response toward other humans. The brain rewards acting on empathy—exercising compassion—by releasing the social bonding hormone oxytocin, which makes us feel warm and caring. A kind act improves the giver's physical health and ability to deal with stress.

In his book, Nichols cites numerous programs aimed at helping people—from wounded vets to drug addicts—who feel whole by engaging with water. A group called Heroes on the Water teaches vets to fish from kayaks with a triple punch of physical, occupational, and mental therapy. Another program, FleaHab, teaches addicts to catch a wave to trade their drug habit for the dopamine rush of a healthful activity. In both these cases, the group nature of the activity fuels cohesion by the release of oxytocin. It also changes the brain's chemistry.

When one considers that the evidence that the modern Western population's divorce from nature and marriage to technology is creating a more narcissistic and selfish society and more anxious, self-absorbed individuals, this empathetic response to nature scenes bears further investigation. Spending time in nature, many studies have shown, makes "us feel more connected to something outside of ourselves, something bigger, more transcendent, and universal," says Nichols—the antithesis of narcissism. We come to know nature and become invested in it. People will only protect what they know and love. If they don't know nature, they won't value it or protect it. Conservationists fear that stressed-out, screen-driven millennials won't care for a planet that seems foreign to them—and the earth and human race will pay the price. And in fact a recent study indicated a drop in concern for the environment since the 1970s.

With a master's degree in economics, Nichols takes a distinctively economic view of conservation. First, he says, "You must understand your product. If you don't understand it, you'll undervalue it and despoil it." He believes that what's missing from the conservation movement is the compelling story of the cognitive, emotional, social, and psychological benefits of water. For instance, those benefits, he claims, should have been factored into the BP damages for the Gulf of Mexico oil spill, but they got no hearing. We may still be years from measuring the monetary value of the benefits of nature, but Nichols and a host of other advocates are eager to modify attitudes toward nature.

Now we have the science to back up claims that a walk in the forest or a dip in the ocean is good medicine, the know-how to put that science into action, and evidence of the positive results worldwide. The human brain has a reciprocal relationship with nature. If we keep our planet healthy, nature's ancient medicine will take care of us.

Twelve-year-old Girl
Grooming an Old Horse

by Frannie Lindsay

And though she has entered the wilderness
of adolescence where she must not love
old things, she rises early, keeping clean

her promise to feed him whatever
he still can eat: one or two pieces
of apple, some herbs to ward off colic;

and to brush him as daybreak stands back up
in his shadow's temperate peace, no choice
except to be the pretty rider who always will wear

the dungarees her mother isn't allowed to wash,
the sweatshirt her brother used as a paint rag,
the boots she wanted every year for Christmas.

—for Karen

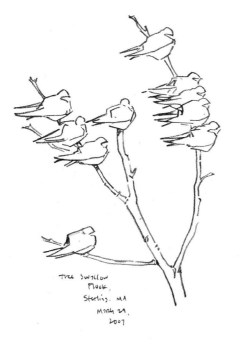

Tree Swallow
Flock,
Sterling, MA
March 29,
2007

The Enduring Animal
The Ancient Roots of Humans' Response to Our Fellow Creatures
by Ron McAdow

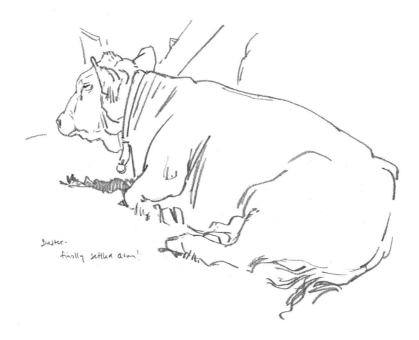

Buster.
finally settled down!

Why is it that birds as well as lions, tigers, and bears mean so much to so many? When did this interest begin, and what, if anything, could this interrelationship mean in terms of human health?

It's clear that our fascination with animals long precedes civilization. More than forty thousand years ago, Paleolithic people created small carvings of animals in ivory and antler, and throughout southern France and northern Spain they decorated the interiors of limestone caverns with drawings, paintings, and engravings. Both of these durable forms, the portable and the cave art, were singularly devoted to animals. They depict bison, mammoths, horses, and other quadrupeds, and the likenesses are accurately proportioned and expressive of the spirited life of the subjects.

The artists favored large mammals. Topping the herbivores, supreme in size at five tons, was the woolly mammoth. Rouffignac Cave in the Dordogne, France, has over 150 images of mammoths; including one known as the Patriarch, a giant mammoth with huge tusks. Woolly rhinoceroses also appear on various cave walls. These massive versions of today's rhinos weighed half as much as mammoths, but they carried their mass low to the ground behind fearsome horns.

Aurochs, the ancestors of domestic cattle, are common on certain cave walls, as are steppe bison, the forebearers of the American bison. Both these animals were huge, weighing about a ton. But along with bears, lions, hyenas, as well as the European cave lions, the animal most frequently depicted in Paleolithic art is the horse, suggesting that it has been a greatly beloved animal for a very long time.

Of the wild horses of the Ice Age steppes, the most frequently painted is Przewalski's horse, which is now limited to Mongolia. Also depicted was the tarpan, the wild species that was later domesticated. Horse images in caves include the group of amazing heads depicted at Chauvet in southern France and also excellent drawings on the Great Ceiling at Rouffignac.

The oldest known Paleolithic art is dated at 32,000 years before present, the product of a culture known as Aurignacian. The latest was made about 12,000 years ago, and the earliest is generally judged by critics to be as good as the last.

But who were the Paleolithic artists and why did they make so many pictures of animals? Investigators have shed a fair amount of light on the first question and very little on the second. The artists were European early modern humans, and were behaviorally basically the same as us. They made musical instruments and long-range plans, and wore jewelry, and even decorated themselves with tattoos. Previous species of hominids, for a half-million years at least, had used fire and made stone tools. Based on their large brains, use of symbols, and complex social organization, the great capacity of the art makers is thought to have been associated with a rich complex spoken language. These Paleolithic people also had fine tools including needles, and well-made fur clothing that was especially important for those living in Ice Age conditions. Although they visited caves, they did not live in them. They made shelters from animal hides, which often were pitched beneath overhanging rock ledges.

The lack of a written record makes it impossible to know exactly why these early Europeans made art. There are numerous lines of thought. The first great authority, Henri Breuil, argued in the early twentieth century that the purpose of the pictures was to improve hunting outcomes. "Everywhere it was big game hunters who produced beautiful naturalistic art," he wrote. He hypothesized that hunters approached prey species by disguising themselves as animals; their artwork reflected a belief that the disguises themselves had magical power. Breuil recognized that the people who created these images had an "artistic temperament and adoration of beauty," and he speculated on the possibilities of songs and other effects to make caves the venues of impressive ceremonies.

Archaeologists have analyzed the campsites of these ancient hunters, some of which were at the mouths of caves, although most were in the open air. The preponderance of reindeer bones suggested that many groups had subsisted largely on that species—but the art the people created emphasized bison and horses, which tends to undercut Breuil's "hunting magic" explanation for the motivation behind the art.

The next generation of experts argued that the early western Europeans were under continuous transformation and that no attempt to understand them should rely on comparison with primitive peoples existing in historic times. They thought it likely that animals represented clans. They analyzed spatial relationships of images and drew associations between species and what they thought of as male and female principles. One researcher, Max Raphael, suggested that the animal pictures symbolized humanity's emergence from, and superiority to, the matrix of zoological life.

More recent theories assert that the artists were tribal shamans trying to reproduce visions they had experienced during trances induced by fasting or drugs. Jean Clottes and David Lewis-Williams expounded this view in *The Shamans of Prehistory*, grounding their argument in neurobiology and ethnology. None of these ideas is without points of interest, but none has found acceptance as a complete explanation for the art. Although we cannot view this art without sensing its precious place in our human heritage, we are left wondering about its original purpose. Because those people had the same nervous system as we do, we have license to speculate how their cultures might have used the pictures. Henri Breuil suggested the possibility of mysterious ceremonies and stories. The oral tales and beliefs of Paleolithic peoples are hidden from us—conjecture we must.

One of the ideas about why they made animal art has an attractive reversibility. The genus *Homo* began as one beast among many, but *Homo sapiens* ascended to a whole new level of dangerousness. Perhaps animal images betray a pride in that preeminence—or maybe on the contrary they result from a longing to identify with our swift, graceful, powerful fellow mammals. The pictures can be read to express envy of the animals' majesty and our aspiration to feel as strong and robust as bison and horses appear to feel. But who knows what solace, or sense of belonging, or physiological benefits these ancient ancestors derived from this deep association with the natural world.

By the nature of the situation, theories about the artworks' purpose cannot be tested. A simple need for self-expression could also be an incentive. Interpreters at the caves usually decline to speculate about the artists' intentions. In the end, the pictures pose more questions than answers. They were obviously spiritual in some way, but beyond that who knows?

As ice retreated and the climate warmed, forests gradually replaced the grassy steppes that had supported huge numbers of meaty herbivores, and from the East came agriculture, wheels, cities, kings, and bureaucracy.

Eden and Eden's animal cave art were finished—but our wish to see and understand and associate with animals has never gone away.

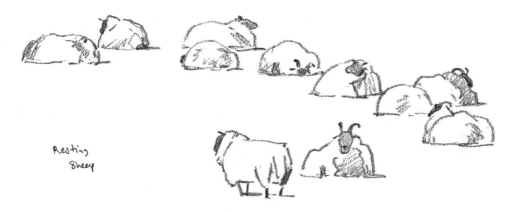

Resting
Sheep

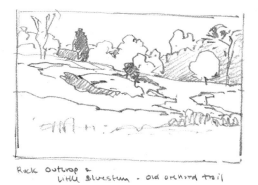

Rock outcrop &
Little Bluestem - Old Orchard trail

A human being may well ask an animal: "Why do you not speak to me of your happiness but only stand and gaze at me?" The animal would like to answer, and say "the reason is I always forget what I was going to say"—but then he forgot this answer too, and stayed silent; so that the human being was left wondering.

–Friedrich Nietzsche, *On the Advantage and Disadvantage of History for Life*

The dog is just about to answer my question

by Frannie Lindsay

except he always forgets
the pithy, rehearsed response he had ready
in perfectly fluent Doglish, his tar-black lips
taking their time to form each *ooo*
And consonant, each virtuoso diphthong,

and then he forgets what I asked him and why,
and now the mother noun and all of her dazed little
adjectives have skittered off into the weeds,
leaving only the scent of their eloquence.
And though his dopily honest eyes

peer in the approximate right direction; although
his ears exclaim about something-or-other; although
he knows a scavenge in dirt is fun—rooting around
for his soggy ball, clamping his dagger-teeth
deep in an unlucky bird shadow;

still, like a great great aunt who can't quite
recall the names of her dinner guests,
he's turning each page of his blissfully colorblind
scrapbook of dreams so he might remember
what fun is, one of these days.

Doctor Dog
The Health Benefits of Humans' Best Friend
by Gayle Goddard-Taylor

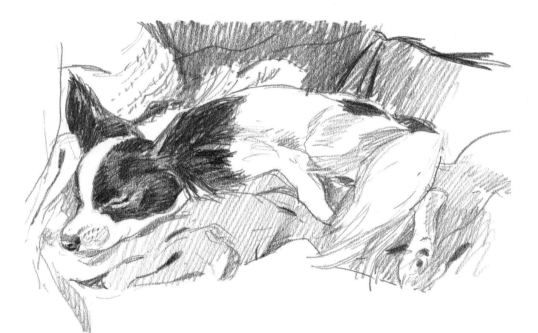

The greyhounds move quietly through the adult day care center, stopping to gently touch nose to hand or rest a muzzle on a knee. They are rewarded with petting and cooing. One of the dogs approaches an old man, hunched in his chair and staring into the long distance. A staff person whispers that the man has been completely unresponsive, failing to initiate or return conversation with anyone in the room, and he will likely ignore the dog.

But the dog knows better. A nuzzle is returned with petting, and the man's eyes begin to focus on the dog.

"My wife and I used to raise German shepherds," he says to no one in particular, and the words begin to flow.

In those few seconds of dog-human interaction, when canine eyes met human eyes and hand touched head, history repeated itself. It might have been something like that, the first tentative reaching out between species that occurred tens of thousands of years ago and ultimately led to the domestic dog.

That animals provide us with a multitude of intangible gifts is no secret. Ask any dog, cat, or horse owner about their beloved pets and a gush of anthropomorphic descriptions of their relationship will ensue. His dog knows when he is sad and tries to cheer him up; the cat knows when she is sick and lies atop her purring soothingly; the horse begins whinnying as soon as, and only when, its owner's car approaches the stable.

Can dogs actually love? Does a cat have a sixth sense about illness? Can a horse really differentiate between car engines? The relationship between humans and animals has long been the subject of novels and movies, but in recent years science is catching up to the fact that our pets do indeed confer health benefits to their human families.

Before the question of how and when those benefits accrue, we need to understand how the closest of interspecies bonds—that of humans and dogs—has evolved over the years. Underlying that bond is the greatest attachment of all, our connection with the natural world that has been shaped by millions of years of living—and learning to survive—within it. This relationship, which evolutionary biologist Edward O. Wilson labeled biophilia in his book of the same name, is imprinted in our neural circuitry. It is why we are, for the most part, fascinated by and tend to gravitate toward other species and natural habitats.

The first creature to actually be domesticated was the wolf—the gray wolf, in particular, from which modern dogs evolved. While the dog's predecessor is no longer in doubt, thanks to DNA evidence, the matter of exactly when, where, and in how many locations the first domestication(s) occurred is the subject of much debate.

In the nineteenth century, the earliest remains of a doglike animal (based on the length of its snout) were discovered in a cave in Belgium and dated to 31,000 years ago. But the archeological record so far showed no more evidence of these creatures until the bones of a similar animal were discovered in western Russia. Carbon dating put these remains somewhere between 12,000 and 14,000 years ago, predating humankind's own transition to agriculture.

In a paper published in 2009, a group of Swedish researchers contended that studies of the mitochondrial DNA of 1,500 dogs point to a single domestication event about 16,300 years ago in China. In an article for *Archeology* (September/October 2010), authors Jarrett A. Lobell and Eric A. Powell reported that archeological evidence suggests that domestications of the dog occurred in multiple locations—and at different times. It is the theory to which John Bradshaw, PhD, biologist and author of *In Defence of Dogs: Why Dogs Need Our Understanding*, subscribes.

"The apparent contradiction between the archaeological evidence and DNA evidence can be reconciled if we posit not just one domestication event, but several, in different parts of the world," Bradshaw writes.

The archeological record isn't all that helpful, however, in pinpointing when humans and dogs began their journey together. Recent discoveries of grave sites in Asia and Europe containing humans and dogs buried together date back 14,000 to 15,000 years. But they don't provide evidence of a "first domestication" event.

Just when enough trust had been built between the two species to overcome suspicion can only be imagined. One theory suggests it happened when the more sociable wolf ventured into a hunting camp to snatch scraps. Another theory, perhaps more plausible, imagines that humans collected and raised the cubs of the more sociable wolf. Cubs may have been selected for their temperaments and would have likely bred with other more tractable wolves until a creature with the temperament and willingness to live among us and serve mankind emerged.

Evidence of one of the earliest ways in which the dog was trained to be of service to humankind is contained on a Roman fresco dating to the first century AD that depicts a dog leading a blind man. In the mid-1700s, guide dogs were trained at a Parisian hospital for the blind, although the modern guide dog movement didn't gain strength until later when, at the end of World War I, thousands of soldiers robbed of their sight by mustard gas returned home. Additional guide dog training schools sprang up across Europe and then spread to the US.

Training a dog to fetch or to navigate for us relies largely on temperament and trainability. Over the past few decades, dogs have expanded their repertoire even further. Researchers from all parts of the globe who have studied the relationships between dogs and their owners have found that stroking the pet or even simply making eye contact causes oxytocin to surge in both pet and owner. That surge has been shown to lead to lowered blood pressure and heart rate in both.

This soothing end product of merely stroking a dog (or cat, horse, or even a guinea pig) is one way in which animals have become, in a sense, health care providers. It has fueled an explosion of studies in a field now known as Human/Animal Interaction (HAI) to further investigate this phenomenon. Even before the relatively recent wave of studies, a variety of animal-assisted therapy programs emerged based on anecdotal evidence.

These days, therapy dogs routinely visit nursing homes and assisted-living complexes to comfort elderly residents and generate more social interaction. At the Cummings School of Veterinary Medicine at Tufts University in Grafton, Massachusetts, researchers have found that owning a dog motivates the elderly to exercise. The six-year-old program, Tufts Paws for People, dispatches certified pet visitation teams to nursing homes, libraries, hospitals, and residential facilities for children with behavioral issues. Paws for People recently partnered with the national Pet Partners, which has strict standards-based requirements for its dogs and handlers. Anecdotal evidence that the soothing presence of a therapy dog is beneficial in a variety of situations is mounting.

"The field of human-animal interaction has really gotten larger over the past 10 years or so," says Megan Mueller, PhD, a psychology professor at Tufts who has carved out a niche in the field of human-animal interaction. "People have been studying it for a while, but it wasn't their primary field. It would be nurses or social workers or pediatricians. Now we're seeing it become a mainstream field, but it's still very interdisciplinary."

Mueller is studying whether an equine-assisted therapy program for adolescents with symptoms of Post Traumatic Stress Disorder (PTSD) can help either through the youths riding, or simply through grooming horses and being in their presence. All the kids in the study are also receiving standard treatments as well. Equine-Assisted Therapy (EAT), while not new, has been the focus in recent years of researchers who want to determine what the most effective treatment modalities are in cases like these.

There also is ongoing research on the effect interacting with animals may have on children diagnosed with the pervasive Attention-Deficit/Hyperactivity Disorder (ADHD). Sabrina Schuck, an assistant clinical professor of pediatrics at UC Irvine, recently concluded a four-year study that examined a group of 8 and 9 year olds with ADHD. The study utilized a certified therapy dog in conjunction with a standard cognitive/behavioral treatment protocol to determine if the dog's presence would reduce the children's symptoms and encourage social skills.

The children were divided into two groups, with both receiving the standard treatment. But only one group was allowed to spend time playing with a therapy dog as a reward for behaving well. The other group was rewarded with cuddle time with a stuffed animal. The dogs were of different breeds, and the study was conducted in 12-week increments with follow-ups done six weeks out. In all, 90 children were part of the study.

"Our main aim was to see if the presence of a dog improved behavior in school and at home for these children," says Schuck. "We also wanted to see if the children gained particular social skills, specifically empathy and reduced bullying and aggressiveness. And we wanted to see if parent-child relationships improved."

While both groups showed a reduction in the symptoms of inattention and hyperactivity, the greatest changes were demonstrated by those children who interacted with a live dog. This group also showed the greatest improvement in social orientation and adaptive social skills. "An interesting finding," Schuck notes, "was that the rate of improvement was faster in the dog group than in the control group and that the gains appeared to hold up—at least in the short-term."

Parents and teachers reported marked improvements in their children's behavior, from sitting still more often to demonstrating greater calmness, both of which allowed the students to focus on the learning challenges at hand. "Perhaps not surprisingly, a number of the families whose children were involved in the study ended up getting a dog," says Schuck.

Anecdotal evidence abounds that veterans with PTSD can benefit greatly from the calming influence of a dog. But because there have been few evidence-based studies that support the premise, the federal Veterans Health Administration does not currently provide service or emotional support dogs to vets suffering from PTSD. It does provide veterinary care for the service dogs of veterans with a permanent disability, however.

The difference between a registered service dog and an emotional support dog is primarily a matter of access. Service dogs are allowed into spaces, such as airplanes and restaurants, that are off-limits for emotional support dogs. For veterans who have found relief through the companionship of a dog, this lack of access can be a significant hardship. But the issue has now come to the fore, both because of the numbers of veterans suffering from PTSD and the champions who advocate for emotional support dogs for them.

Butch and Theresa Bouchard, both PTSD sufferers after serving in the

Canadian military, don't need an evidence-based study to tell them that having a therapy dog means the difference between a life spent in fear of leaving the house and a life lived to the fullest. Butch suffered from severe PTSD after serving in the pirate-infested waters off the coast of Africa. His sleep was interrupted by horrific nightmares; he perpetually fidgeted and frequently overreacted to everyday occurrences. He was also unwilling to leave the house without his wife by his side.

"The military is very good at teaching you to function when you're at a very high stress level," says Butch, "but then you have no switch to turn it off."

The Bouchard's marriage had reached a crisis point by the time they heard about therapy dogs through Luis Carlos Montalván, a highly decorated veteran and author of the best-selling book *Until Tuesday*. Montalván, who suffered from PTSD before acquiring his dog, Tuesday, now travels the country with his dog, advocating for veterans and assistance dogs.

Not long after meeting Montalván, the Bouchards adopted Skittles, a rescued Australian shepherd puppy, and Butch's nightmares soon began to disappear, his fidgeting decreased, and the pair could be seen all around town—without Theresa in tow. Then, the worst happened. The young dog died on the operating table as she was being anesthetized for spaying. Her death sent Butch into a downward spiral. But a breeder in British Columbia heard about his plight and offered a pup from a recent litter. The new companion, Spirit of Grace, took up her post with enthusiasm. But the family's tortured journey through the complicated world of service dog training and government regulation transformed them into advocates for emotional support dogs.

Spirit has provided Butch with the needed "off-switch." Whether she is sensing his elevating heartbeat or detecting the chemicals produced in his brain, she will nudge him with her nose or pull on the leash to divert him from whatever he is hyperfocusing upon.

"When she does that," says Theresa, "she's preventing him from having an anxiety or panic attack."

Here in the US, the matter of dogs for PTSD sufferers was tackled from a different angle by service dog trainer Rick Yount, who established a unique school at a VA hospital in Menlo Park, California. In 2008, Yount recruited 200 vets with PTSD and trained them, in turn, to train service dogs for disabled vets. It was a stroke of genius. Vets who feared revealing they suffered from PTSD were more than willing to participate in a program to help fellow soldiers. The program was well received, turned out properly trained service dogs, and led to a career as accredited service dog trainers for two of the veteran-trainers.

Yount presented his findings at the 2009 Veterans Mental Health Conference and the annual meeting of the International Society for Traumatic Stress Studies. Yount reported that veteran-trainers demonstrated improvements in a variety of areas, including increased patience, impulse control, and emotional regulation and decreased depression, pain perception, and startle response. Their communication skills also improved, as did their sleep behavior, and a positive sense of purpose emerged.

Since then, 3,000 service members and veterans have gone through Yount's voluntary Warrior Canine Connection program at "Healing Quarters" in Brookeville, Maryland. But there still remains the need for science-based evidence that would convince the VA and insurers to provide financial assistance for costly training. To that end, Yount and author Meg Daley Olmert, who wrote *Made for Each Other: The Biology of the Human-Animal Bond*, have partnered on a small government-funded pilot program, the Warrior Canine Connection study, which will involve 40 vets with PTSD.

According to Olmert, the science on oxytocin has been done; she believes that oxytocin is working its magic for vets. "PTSD is a very complex disorder that has neurochemical, behavioral, and sleep-interruption effects. Basically, the veteran is stuck in 'fight-or-flight' mode. The only thing that will turn that off is oxytocin."

Each veteran-trainer in the Warrior Canine Connection pilot will work with the young dogs for two weeks at a time. Before and after each session, the veteran's levels of neurochemicals, including oxytocin, will be measured. Also gauged will be a range of the psychological symptoms of PTSD. All measures will be rechecked at six months and again a year after the program concludes.

"The genius of this is that the training of the dog is the medicine," says Olmert. "The veteran with PTSD is willing to participate (as the trainer of the pup) because he's knows he's helping a fellow veteran in need. The science is that this kind of training and nurturing of the dog releases oxytocin in the brain and body of the vet with PTSD. It's a win–win."

If neurochemicals are the elixir at the bottom of all of the aforementioned therapies, it is the dog's extraordinary physiology that is at work in the numerous other ways dogs warn us, protect us, diagnose life-threatening health concerns, and even protect the environment. We are talking about the dog's nose, which seems to detect scent out of thin air—and, in fact, does.

Biologist-author John Bradshaw explains that at some point in the past primitive humans had more acute olfactory abilities than we have today. Over the millennia, the part of the brain devoted to odor detection shrank in order to make room for expanding human vision to include color detection. Canines, on the other hand, evolved into far more advanced scent detectors, a skill they apparently found more useful.

"We have complicated color vision so it's been a trade-off," says Bradshaw. "Dogs and humans together are the best of both worlds."

Tucked away in Alabama is an unusual program that is devoted to exploring and utilizing the dog's olfactory talents. The Canine Performance Sciences Program at Auburn University's College of Veterinary Medicine has a mission statement that says it all—"the continuing improvement of animal detection science through research and technology to serve the nation and society." The program has gained international recognition for its dogs and the tasks they undertake.

"We utilize dogs as a mobile sensory tool in a variety of ways," says Craig Angle, associate director of Canine Performance Sciences. "Anything you want to detect, we devise ways to have dogs detect it—explosives, viruses, microscopic fungi growing underground. It's really amazing what the dogs' capabilities are."

And just how far do those capabilities extend? Beginning with the nose itself, science now knows that dogs can detect scents that are in the parts per trillion, although it is suspected it doesn't stop there—it's just that the tool to accurately measure anything smaller has yet to be invented. A Labrador retriever's nose contains as many as 300 million sensory receptors spread across 30 square inches of surface area that is configured in numerous folds. The human nose, by comparison, has about 5 to 6 to million receptors. The amount of the canine brain devoted to olfaction is roughly 30 to 40 times that of the human brain.

"A large part of why they detect smells so well has to do with fluid dynamics and how air flows through the dog's nose," says Angle. "They are able to separate the air that comes in so that about 12 to 13 percent goes to the olfactory tissue and the rest goes into the lungs."

Over the years, Auburn has developed its own breeding program to come up with a dog that has not only superior scent detection but is highly motivated to put its nose to work. The breed, which has no real name, is largely from Labrador retriever lines that have shown exceptional detection traits. Pups spend their first year of life, like any other dog, learning to be a good citizen but are also being evaluated for behavioral traits, trainability, and intelligence. "It's amazing to see," says Angle. "These dogs don't want to retrieve or even be petted. They just want to work the air currents and the environment."

The trained dogs are placed with clients around the world for a variety of scent-detection jobs. While the "bread and butter" of the Auburn program has always been its explosives-trained dogs, more recent uses to which these specialized canine noses are being put have been nothing short of astonishing. In recent years, these dogs have been put to work resolving some thorny environmental issues.

The bumblebees of Scotland, which are under siege by an as-yet-unidentified

Outside In
Bringing the Natural World to People Confined Indoors
by Thomas Conuel

In the spring of 1889, an ailing Vincent Van Gogh came to the asylum of Saint Paul de Mausole in Saint-Rémy-de-Provence, France, seeking succor from the mental and emotional storms that tore at him. Inspired by the natural beauty of the place, especially the asylum's gardens where he spent days wandering and studying the shapes of flowers, Van Gogh began painting assiduously—producing in a short time 130 paintings including *Irises*, a now-famous portrait of blue irises with a single white iris in their midst, and orange flowers in the background; a rendering often considered a tribute to the healing powers of nature that soothed the artist at the time.

Van Gogh was hardly the first to find peace, insight, and creative growth in nature. Henry Thoreau found similar sustenance some 44 years earlier, living and writing on the shores of Walden Pond as he tried to find solace after the death of his brother, John. Scores of seekers have followed in his footsteps since, often substituting a slice of backyard greenery behind the garage for Walden Pond or the garden in Provence. Both Van Gogh and Thoreau were able to move about freely on the grounds and woods of their sanctuaries, seeking their own bonds with nature and finding in the natural world a bridge to fulfillment. But what of others who stymied by age, infirmities, or mental or physical disabilities cannot reach out to hug nature on their own?

That was the conundrum that led to founding of The Nature Connection in Concord, in 1983, with a mission to bring the healing power of nature to those who cannot find it without assistance. Originally known as Animals as Intermediaries, The Nature Connection travels bringing educational and therapeutic nature programs, biweekly or monthly, to hospitals, residential schools, at-risk youth programs, special-needs facilities, nursing homes, and

Alzheimer's care programs. All places where the residents are mostly confined inside.

Stop by the offices of The Nature Connection, two rooms in the back of a stately three-story brick building near Concord Center, and talk with Sophie Wadsworth, a poet, teacher, the executive director of The Nature Connection since 2010, and a member of the staff since 2008. In the back room, Sophie will show you the "ocean context box," a small container with a layer of sand, pebbles, and seashells inside. Tilt it back and forth and listen to the sound—like waves on the seashore; it's useful for starting conversations about the ocean and the many creatures that call it home. The room is full of other context boxes and jars containing herbs, spices, gourds, dried flowers—and all evoke memories.

Of course, there are the animals too, the perennial stars of every visit from The Nature Connection. They stay at the homes of various volunteer caregivers and include dogs and cats, owls and crows, hawks and robins, chickens and baby chicks, doves and ducks, rabbits and guinea pigs, and assorted catch-and-release tadpoles, toads, and turtles. On The Nature Connection website, the menagerie is listed as "current staff or visiting professors." (Those volunteers who keep wild animals do so as federal- and state-licensed wildlife handlers.)

Dogs, cats, and guinea pigs have comforted the sick, the elderly, and the disabled for many decades, but duplicating a slice of wild nature for therapeutic effects is a relatively new concept. The Nature Connection programs change with the seasons: perhaps a meadow in autumn, a salt marsh in winter, or the edge of a forest between suburbia and the wild in spring. The idea remains the same: bring the essence of a natural place to those who cannot get there on their own. "We bring nature; nature does the rest," is the guiding principle.

On a typical site visit, staff and volunteers wheel carts loaded with buckets and jars filled with treasures from a morning natural history ramble—a pinecone, a tadpole, an oak leaf, an acorn. They push through hospital lobbies, nursing home entrances, and locked juvenile facilities to introduce those inside to the healing power of natural associations and to "gently transform the institutional setting with a sense of the wild," says Sophie Wadsworth.

During a program, a volunteer might talk about the cycle of life and ask how seeds find their way to the right place where they can sprout into plants and trees, or how a snowy winter provides an inward resting time for plants and animals following the abundance of spring and summer. There are stories and songs, and reaching out, asking for others to share their own narratives.

At a hospital school serving young children, the volunteers "build" a meadow—placing on the floor a large canvas mat or two and then grasses, rocks, soil, logs, pine needles, cattails, pumpkins, gourds, grapevines, and a rabbit. All treasures from a walk through a meadow that morning, except the rabbit who resides with a volunteer at The Nature Connection. The children ask questions and appoint themselves as caretakers of the rabbit. "He needs a place to hide," notes one child. Others move grasses and sticks around to create a nest for the rabbit.

At another site on another day, a group of boys gathers to first watch and then hold a five-foot gopher snake, in the process overcoming their own fears of snakes and learning to work together to safely hold and not drop the large and writhing reptile. A few moments later, a small screech-owl perches on a hand as the instructor points out how the owl rotates its head in a near full circle.

In a classroom full of teenagers in wheelchairs, Suzanne, a staff member, brings a barred owl with a missing wing. The noise and disruptions stop and the questions begin. Will the owl ever fly again? How does it eat? Can it grow another wing? Several of the teenagers are missing limbs of their own. Suzanne explains that the owl's wing will never grow back, but that the owl has grown strong in other ways, using her tail for balance to compensate for the missing wing, becoming extra vigilant when strange creatures approach. The owl hops about on the ground. She has adapted to her injury and survives. It is a lesson for the teenagers, one of whom looks at her missing hand and then at the owl.

At yet another site, this one for the elderly, many suffering from memory loss, a woman sits alone, refusing to participate in the afternoon's program. But then somebody offers her a gourd to touch. She turns away, but then after a moment turns back. Slowly she reaches out to touch the gourd. This, she says, speaking for the first time in months, reminds her of her youth and her family's farm, and the deepening autumn days, and the gourds her family gathered for Halloween. She smiles.

It is a tenet of The Nature Connection that, while animals enhance and illustrate the program, the same draw toward nature and the great cycle of life on earth can happen as someone looks at and holds a rock or a leaf. A maple leaf on the ground in autumn evokes the closing of a yearly cycle—the seasons change and go round. Living things bloom and flourish and then die. Winter comes, but spring follows. The maple tree must prepare for winter, but it will once again be green.

Dogs are always popular and help build trust, serving as an "excellent reference"—as they bring assurance with their trust and love that we, the people with the dog, are good people. And like all animals they are nonjudgmental; they don't pull back from a person who cannot speak or is missing a leg or a hand.

The origins of The Nature Connection go back to the early 1970s and the holistic philosophy that inspired many educators at the time. Sarah Reynolds and Nancy Mattila collaborated with several other teachers to start the School for Centered Learning in Concord that, among other accomplishments, created a traveling educational, therapeutic arts, and nature program. Since then The Nature Connection has taken as its mission the task of bringing the natural world to those who cannot find it on their own.

Sarah Reynolds's daughter, Rebecca Reynolds Weil, worked with her mother and served as executive director from 1993 to 2002. Rebecca documented the work of The Nature Connection and its successes in her award-winning book *Bring Me the Ocean: Nature as Teacher, Messenger, and Intermediary,* which tells the stories of the powerful relationship between those in need and the natural world.

The Nature Connection is growing—300 individuals at eight sites in 2015, but with a vision that foresees site visits spreading across Massachusetts, including pilot programs that will "teach the teacher" and help spread The Nature Connection mission.

In *Bring Me the Ocean*, Rebecca Reynolds Weil describes an encounter with a disabled man with a strange request: "Bring me the ocean," requested Jim. But how does one transport the ocean to a severely disabled patient who suffered a traumatic head injury that left him as a triplegic unable to speak? All Jim's language-based interaction occurs by way of a communication board on the armrest of his wheelchair.

After a second request from Jim, Suzanne asked Jim, "How should we bring you the ocean?" And Jim replied, "in buckets." The staff thought about that and on their next visit brought buckets full of water from the Atlantic and other buckets with seaweed, mussels, clams, periwinkles, and a lobster. Jim, it turned out, had been a lobsterman before his incapacitating injury, and had spent much of his adult life at sea. He wanted to see, smell, and feel the ocean around him once again.

"A past emerged," writes Weil, "and Jim showed us that anything, even the ocean, can be brought into an institution. Over the years, requests such as Jim's have extended the scope of our programs, encouraging us to expand our own perception of what is possible." ❧

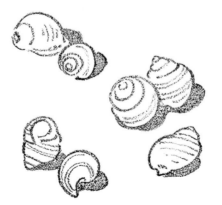

Ephemera

by Margot Wizansky

Just as the raspberries reach
their fragile fullness, and I've
armored myself, leather-gloved,
to pick among thorns, the wasps
beat me to them. I'm a voyeur—
the way the wasps take the berries—
each wasp a little cameo on deep red,
sucking the drupelets, juices dripping,
berry disintegrating—brazen feast!
It aches with beauty, this momentary
life, whether or not we use it well,
it plays us, like that old joke on me:
gift-wrapped box after box,

ribboned and glittered, nested
one inside the other, all empty,
even the last box—only the world
dangling before me, sparkling fine.

The Garden of Earthly Cures
Medicinal Plants Past, Present, and Future
by Teri Dunn Chace

How do plants help humans heal? A botanist, an ethnobotanist, a practicing herbalist, plant geneticist, native healer, or practitioner of ayurvedic or traditional Chinese medicine would all have varying answers to this question, each viewed through the lens of their respective fields. But the short answer is that plants contain compounds that ward off predators and infectious bacteria, fungi, and viruses. Apply topically or ingest certain plants and one may benefit from these same compounds. In effect, when we use plant-based medicinals, we are leveraging the plant's version of an immune system for our own benefit.

While it's not possible to know precisely when people first started using plants for medicinal purposes, suffice to say it's been a very long time. Some archeological research traces the beginnings back to 3700 BC Egypt. The inhabitants of China were also pioneers, as were the early Greeks and Romans. The earliest written accounts of herbal remedies are Chinese and date back to 2800 BC. Here in North America, there is also an extensive history of use of native plants to help and heal, but there are no written records.

Perhaps this is stating the obvious, but before anyone understood how or why plants worked, they were still used and used effectively, although occasionally a patient may have been harmed. Inevitably, local knowledge of regional plants was shared and circulated even before anything was written down, so early healers did not have to keep reinventing the wheel. Knowledge of human anatomy and systems, as well as body chemistry and genetics, has advanced remarkably—and continues to—but this does not necessarily mean that primitive plant medicine was ineffective. For instance, willow water, made by soaking twigs or bark in water, has long been used everywhere willow trees grow as an anti-inflammatory. Modern science later identified the presence of the glycoside salicin in the willow plants, which became the basis of the little white aspirin pill. Those who initially discovered this use didn't know the precise scientific reason, nor did they need to.

Accessing the useful parts of a plant has also been an area for exploration historically. Mint settles an upset stomach best when dried leaves have been infused in hot water to make a tea. Eating purple coneflower to access the plant's antibiotic or immune-system-boosting benefits isn't very effective; but powdering the dried roots or, better yet, making a tincture is. Tinctures, infused oils, salves, and poultices are additional ways we extract or maximize a plant's healing properties.

An overview of herbal medicine produced by the University of Maryland Medical Center makes another interesting point. "Researchers found that people in different parts of the world tended to use the same or similar plants for the same purposes." Hence the widespread use of willow water, as mentioned before. This would seem to support claims made about the efficacy of many common plants used to treat sick or injured patients.

How is such synchronicity possible? If you ask, the healers in communities far from one another often reply that they *sensed* the proper use, as though it were a matter of intuition or instinct. Some even say that the plant *told* them. Interestingly, this explanation is also often given for how humans have discerned which plants are good or safe to eat. Before we dismiss such explanations, bear in mind that healers past and present study nature carefully in ways that most of us do not.

Since illness and disease have not been eradicated in our modern world, the research continues. In fact, there is a growing sense of urgency because the natural world is so severely threatened by habitat destruction, climate change, and species loss. For all we know, there may be a singular rainforest plant, or a tundra plant, that holds the key to treating all cancers. In the past, medicines derived from the plants of the garden, fields, and forests were not only considered legitimate, but were the primary option. In fact, this is still true in many places in the world, particularly rural Africa and India. The World Health Organization estimates that 80 percent of people worldwide rely on herbal medicines for some part of their primary health care.

There's no denying that over time mainstream Americans began to trust whatever was in the little orange plastic medicine bottle with the printed label more than whatever was growing just outside the door. Significant and innovative medical and pharmaceutical advances have been lifesavers. Yet, in a bid to find effective and/or more affordable alternatives, or perhaps as a backlash, some people have turned (or returned) to herbal medicine and homeopathy.

Claims that "natural medicines" are in general safer or have fewer side effects are not conclusive, however. For example, clinical studies have found that the herbal remedy St. John's Wort interferes with the effectiveness of many drugs, including the blood thinner warfarin (Coumadin), protease inhibitors for HIV, birth control pills, certain asthma drugs, antidepressant pills, and many other medications. On the other hand, numerous laboratory studies confirm that *Ginkgo biloba* improves blood circulation by dilating blood vessels and reducing the stickiness of blood platelets, though it too interferes with Coumadin. In other words, it's hard to generalize.

It is also important to note that the FDA regulates the medications commonly prescribed and purchased in the United States. It's not true that herbs and supplements are totally unregulated. For them, the FDA enforces GMP, or Good Manufacturing Procedures. Some people feel this is insufficient, and quality and claims vary—bad or ineffective products can give the whole field a bad name. Americans interested in exploring herbal medicine are well advised to proceed with caution. Your best bet would be to consult with a qualified experienced herbalist or naturopath.

Plants have consistently proven to be resources important to our survival. Even when we don't quite understand why or how, there is no reason to think we've reached the limit of their potential. The fact is, a great many plant medicines and remedies do work and certainly have stood the test of time. Pharmaceutical companies know this, and part of their research and development continues to probe folk and indigenous knowledge.

A recent trip to a local historic museum reminded me of the journey plant medicines have taken in this country. I was at the Farmer's Museum in Cooperstown, New York. While my husband browsed the many old-fashioned and ingenious farm tools in the huge barn building, I visited a small apothecary hut where a man in period costume was holding forth on colonial-era medicine for the tourists. Presiding over a weathered wooden counter, he deftly rolled up small dried ginger pills while he talked about the sorts of medicines people used over 200 years ago in this part of the world. Ginger's ability to ease digestion and alleviate nausea is well established, and the small group did not look skeptical. Some even accepted his offer to sample one.

I looked around the space, observing jars of dried plants and seeds, mortars and pestles, sieves, and antique bottles and vials. Bundles of herbs hung from the low rafters. There was a shelf of old reference books. In short, it looked to be a thoughtful and authentic reproduction. I was puzzled by something, but I waited until everyone else filed out.

Then we struck up a conversation, and, once he discerned my knowledge of plants and herbs, he dropped out of character. After I complimented him on his ginger-pill presentation, I asked my question: "Ginger is an Old World plant. Didn't the early Americans use native plants for medicine?"

He explained that—as with their food—the first settlers tended to prefer plants they already knew, bringing familiar remedies across the sea from Europe to the new land. This would have included plants such as plantain (the crushed leaves ease the pain or itching of insect bites and rashes), feverfew (leaves infused in tea or eaten in small amounts treated the pain of arthritis and migraine headaches), and mints (for digestive issues). You are likely to see these non-native plants included in the restored gardens of colonial-era interpretive museums from Strawberry Banke in Portsmouth, New Hampshire, to Plimoth Plantation and Sturbridge Village in Massachusetts, to Colonial Williamsburg in Virginia, and they were growing outside the door of the Cooperstown apothecary as well. The efficacy of those Old World plants was established centuries ago and still holds today.

If early white settlers couldn't grow their favorites—and ginger is a tropical plant that our Northeast winters would promptly kill—they'd simply import them. In the book *Jane Colden: America's First Woman Botanist*, the biographer describes the arrival of Jane's father to Philadelphia in 1710. He'd been trained in medicine in Edinburgh, Scotland: "Like other Europeans coming to America, Colden was amazed at how different the New World's flora and fauna was.... He soon became interested in learning about American plants and especially their medicinal applications.... But the need to earn a living prevented him from pursuing his interests right away." He turned to importing medicines.

So, can we gather that although the rich native flora did not go unnoticed by white Europeans, it went unexplored or underutilized? For how long? The Cooperstown apothecary docent showed me a worn, fragile volume entitled *The Dispensatory of the United States of America* (1883), essentially an early herbal, a descriptive catalog of plants and their uses. Garlic, stinging nettle, St. John's wort, mint, chamomile, plantain, cloves, arnica. No surprises here and, at a glance, no especially odd or illegitimate uses, even by modern standards.

But I thumbed through the old book again: no Native American plants; no jewelweed, no witch hazel, no yaupon holly, no evening primrose. Why not? Were the settlers hesitant to use native plants medicinally? Didn't they ask or go to native healers? Or did they feel their own remedies were sufficient?

His opinion was that they were fearful. The American wilderness contained lots of unfamiliar plants. The native people and animals were not always friendly. "It took time to get curious, and comfortable," he opined. In time, the white people did wade in and begin to forage for or grow useful native plants. A book published in 1892, titled *The Cottage Physician: Best Known Methods of Treatment of all Diseases, Accidents and Emergencies at Home*, was by "an intrepid British botanist" who traveled widely throughout the Northeast, gathering and compiling information. By then, the Native American tribes of the Northeast were greatly diminished. When war and territorial conflicts were not the issue, disease was—smallpox, a white man's disease that killed thousands and for which there was no native plant medicine.

In Jane Colden's story, I find another possible reason why native plants didn't make it to the early American apothecary shelves quickly. With her father's encouragement and mentoring, and later correspondence with prominent botanists of the day (John Bartram, Peter Collinson), she produced a fairly extensive American herbal during the years 1753 to 1758. In a book called *Science in the British Colonies in America*, Raymond Phineas Stearns remarked that "[Colden's] plant descriptions were often good, and she displayed a housewifely concern for the uses of plants in cookery and as household remedies for sickness."

Jane evidently consulted other colonial women in her area for that information. Where those women gained the knowledge is an area for speculation. It's also entirely possible they gleaned some information from Native American healers in the region; sometimes such healers were women.

Bear in mind that in the early days of the American colonies, there were myriad cultural exchanges and trade between the white settlers and native people. In a booklet produced by the Smithsonian to accompany a 1980 traveling exhibit *Medicinal Plants in American Indian Life*, ethnobotanist Barrie Kavasch hastens to point out that: "Herbal traditions of every American Indian cultural group on this continent reach far back into prehistory.... [They] had an exceptional understanding of laxative, diuretic, emetic, birth control, and fever-reducing drugs derived from native plants."

Still, a century, or more, was a long time to resist using or mainstreaming native medicinals. Fear of the unknown and other factors could have conspired to keep newcomers from fully discovering and using the extensive body of knowledge that those native to this land had accumulated. Setting aside the social and political issues of the day, we can rue that valuable information was probably lost.

The belief that modern and packaged (and often expensive) medication and treatment is "good," and old-fashioned and homegrown are "bad" or at least risky, bears examination.

Consider this: a Boston friend of mine suffering from ovarian cancer kept the disease's advance at bay for two years with an experimental gene-therapy medication so cutting edge that it is not yet approved by the FDA. Meanwhile, a cancer patient in the Amazon River Basin might be treated by a native healer using the culture's own plant-based medications. It's not easy to say which treatment is superior or which cancer patient is more fortunate because there are so many variables in the treatment of any disease or any specific patient. But we should keep an open mind.

Pharmaceutical firms prefer synthetics or semisynthetics to plants and their derivatives. A sobering study of modern pharmaceuticals done at Purdue University in the early 1990s noted, "25 percent of modern prescription drugs contain at least one compound now or once derived or patterned after compounds derived from higher plants."

What accounts for this low number? It is not merely that old-time herbal medicine has been outpaced or discredited. Part of the answer is that the drug companies want proprietary products. That's where the market share is and, yes, the profit. They may also defend these proportions by saying it is better to manufacture the compounds than strip a forest or field of the useful plants. I'd wager that they find the synthetics cheaper and easier to produce. If a plant offering breakthrough medical benefits could be brought into cultivation one way or another, to create sufficient supply and to deliver consistent uniform harvests—in a profitable and efficient approach—they'd be on it.

There's another practical reason, too. It is often difficult to identify and isolate the part of a plant that provides the sought-after or reputed benefit. To make a medicine, modern lab scientists aim to get at that single active compound. "Trying to find the part of a plant that has a specific effect can be like disassembling a radio to search for the one part that makes the sound," lamented a *National Geographic* article published in 2000 entitled "Nature's Rx." Even the native healer who uses a plant and gets the desired effects may not really know, or know at the level the pharmaceutical researcher wants to know.

Perhaps the active ingredient cannot be isolated easily or work in concert with other compounds also present in a given plant. Consider that there is a synergy that cannot be measured or captured by scientific methods. Each human patient presents a unique body chemistry; each specimen of a plant also presents a unique chemistry. Native healers and traditional herbalists cope with and evaluate based on a gestalt of variables. Isolating an active compound may be neither safe nor desirable. The challenge is that nature is inherently variable. Effects and effectiveness can vary from one specimen of a plant to another, or from one season to another, or from one region to another. Even the properties of one plant may vary.

The fact remains, a wealth of knowledge and potential are still available in nature—this is not hypothetical. There has to be some economic incentive for drug firms to investigate natural alternatives—widespread established ones as well as ones yet to be discovered. If there is a way to patent plants or their compounds and still ensure profits, pharmaceutical companies will find it. My point is that the major drug companies keep an open mind, though not always or exclusively for altruistic reasons.

Virgin American wilderness has long since gone under the plow or been paved over. Pockets of indigenous landscapes and the cultures that inhabit them in remote areas are today's equivalent. Their healers may know things about their plants that can help us all.

The Central and South American jungles, the scrub and desert habitats of Africa and Australia, isolated islands such as Madagascar, and alpine plants worldwide—these are among the present-day areas of interest. Habitat destruction is only part of this race against time. The other peril is equally urgent, the threat of fading and lost knowledge. In the introduction to Mark Plotkin's *Tales of a Shaman's Apprentice: An Ethnobotanist Searches for New*

Medicines in the Amazon Rain Forest, Richard Evans Schultes ticks off the many factors. "Civilization is on the march in many, if not most, primitive regions," he writes. "The rapid divorcement of primitive peoples from dependence upon their immediate environment for the necessities and amenities of life has been set in motion, and nothing will check it now. One of the first aspects of primitive culture to fall before the onslaught of civilization is knowledge and use of plants for medicine. The rapidity of this disintegration is frightening…" Plotkin's book came out in 1993. Schultes' warning is old news.

Back in the September 1988 issue of *Sanctuary* magazine, in the article "Don Eligio's Pharmacy," Rosita Arvigo shared her own challenges in approaching a knowledgeable Mayan shaman in rural Belize. Although she was patient and respectful, although she had demonstrated credentials in botany and herbal medicine, and although she was permitted to help him on his farm and on harvesting expeditions, the elderly healer "evaded the main issue, insisting it was no good to teach a *gringa*." She persisted because she believed his knowledge—part of a long tradition of healers—was precious and important. She was able to get the backing of the New York Botanical Garden and, eventually, to use what she learned and tried to learn in a National Cancer Institute program "to scour the tropical rain forests in search of medicinal plants to be tested against cancer, AIDS, and other diseases."

But you can see the scope of the challenge: the interested foreigner, Arvigo, was just one person, working with one elderly native healer, in a small geographic area. As Plotkin perceptively said, "Every time one of these medicine men dies before someone can capture his knowledge, it is as though an entire library has burned down." Indigenous knowledge frequently is transmitted orally, person to person, mentor to student, while the Western world seeks written recorded data and information.

A case in point is soursop, or graviola, *Annona muricata*. A relative of the paw paw, it's a broadleaf evergreen tree that grows in South and Central America and many Caribbean islands as well as parts of tropical Africa and Asia. Its fruit is long, green, and prickly; inside there's edible white pulp and black seeds. With a hint of sour citrus, the fruit is popular in drinks and desserts. Traditionally, soursop has been used as a way to fight infection and chronic disease. As a cancer treatment, it is said to target only malignant cells, though claims of it being "10,000 times more effective than chemotherapy" seem beyond belief.

Memorial Sloan-Kettering's Cancer Center relegates it to a "purported" treatment, while Cancer Research UK states that "in laboratory studies, graviola extracts can kill some types of liver and breast cancer cells that are resistant to particular chemotherapy drugs. But there haven't been any large-scale studies in humans…so we do not support the use of graviola to treat cancer."

Efforts to gather information leading to the creation of a profitable medication brought on another problem, an ethical one: the issue of intellectual property. Are medical researchers and big pharmaceutical companies getting away with helping themselves to and profiting from indigenous knowledge and plants? The answer seems to be "not so much" in recent times. In 2007, scientists sat down with local healers in Kenya to try to hammer out an agreement.

The policy, which will eventually become law, lays out a strategy to conserve traditional plants, which often are overharvested in the wild, establish the safety and efficacy of traditional remedies, and commercialize remedies on the world market. It also addresses intellectual property, primarily to ensure that traditional healers are compensated for drugs that are eventually sold. Specifically, the agreement states that before scientists can start work, documents must be signed so profits are shared if drugs are developed.

"The existing IP [intellectual property] rights mechanism doesn't contain enough provisions to protect traditional medicine," said Jack Kaguo Githae, a traditional healer from Central Kenya who has contributed to the consultation. "We need to develop an African solution. Benefit sharing is very important. It is a communal resource, and I think it should be approached like that."

Through this agreement, implemented in 2013, the precedents are set. Other examples cited in a report by the World Intellectual Property Organization (WIPO) include a recent agreement between traditional healers in Samoa for a share of the benefit from an AIDS drug that drew upon their knowledge of the mamala tree. The Kani tribe of South India now shares in the benefits of a new sports drug that is based on their knowledge of the medicinal plant arogyapacha. And so on.

Let's hope any and all plant-based remedies will be made available to those who can benefit from them. Therein lies the advantage of outsiders coming in to gather material and information for scientific research and potentially wider distribution. ❧

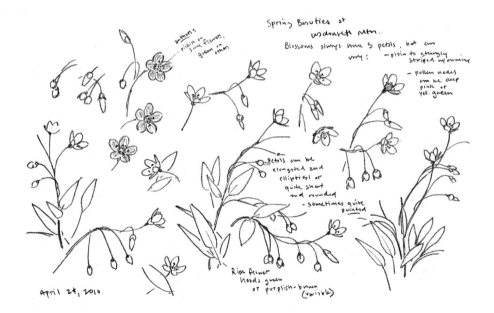

Runways

by Moira Linehan

They dined on mince and slices of quince,
which they ate with a runcible spoon.
–Edward Lear, "The Owl and the Pussycat"

A child's running commentary, a runnel's
nonsense mouthings strung out in tongue-long lines
of bubbles around every tree trunk, log jam,
boulder in the way, then brung back into pools
and eddies, drunken delight at whatever's there,
each ounce wrung out, wrung out. Then abandoned
as children do. Now runic, the allure
of white rocks flattened by the brunt force
of glaciers as they trundled through. In shallows,
in runny mud along banks, along paths
through pine woods, those shining stones runways
to where children dine with runcible spoons.

Two Haiku

by Brad Bennett

half a moon
high above
a quiet cove

swamp morning glory . . .
since the beginning
of time

The Heart of the Matter
by Thomas Conuel

In first grade, I attended a parochial school run by an order of fierce nuns. Sister Agnes Marie, the first-grade teacher, was not one to coddle students. Perhaps a month into the semester, she was delivering a lecture to the boys in the class—the girls had gone to another classroom for their own admonishments—and a dozen bigger boys from higher grades had been brought into our classroom to hear Sister's talk. Sister Agnes Marie would not tolerate impure thoughts and desires in any boy. These were the work of the devil, and boys were particularly prone to his horrid enticements. I had not the faintest idea what she was talking about, but managed to maintain a frozen look of concentration while not fidgeting and sitting ramrod straight in my chair. She was reminding us of her determination to stamp out these vile manifestations of Satan's handiwork when she spied the large muscular boy next to me smirking.

"Wipe that smile off your face, Mr. Dermody," she intoned, "or I shall wipe it off for you."

Dermody was slow to comply so Sister Agnes Marie strode purposefully to her desk where she kept a wicker basket full of tennis balls. I had noticed the basket from the first day of class and wondered why a nun kept tennis balls on her desk. Seizing a ball, she pivoted and fired it across the room with a powerful, accurate throw that a major league baseball player would be proud of, winging it off Dermody's right ear. The tennis ball caromed around the room, and Dermody stopped smiling, looked befuddled and then baffled, and then bit his lip to stop from crying. I had been afraid of Sister Agnes Marie before; now I was terrified.

I had started the school year badly anyhow. Every morning on the school bus I would ask my older brother, Bruce, who was in charge of shepherding me to and from school, the same question several times on the ride.

"How long is the school day?" I would ask him

"Six hours," he would reply.

I would wait several minutes, and then again.

"Bruce, how long is the school day?"

"Six hours."

And again. And yet again.

At the age of six, I was due for open-heart surgery and had missed many days of school because of appointments with heart doctors. As a result, I was afraid of doctors, hospitals, teachers, and school. Doctors probed and scrutinized me. Adults looked at me as if I were about to come apart before their eyes. School made me nervous. I was afraid of the ride on the school bus; I was afraid of Sister Agnes Marie; I was afraid of not completing my homework correctly; I was afraid of entering the confessional booth and reciting my sins to the priest. I was afraid of everything, except the woods.

I spent most of my free time outdoors, alone, wandering a woodlot behind my house in a newly constructed suburb in the Berkshires. It was the only way I had to escape the turmoil of my life before and after the surgery. Outside of school, in the woods, I was not afraid.

My woods was a mix of pine and hardwoods on perhaps 35 acres that had probably been clear-cut once in the late nineteenth-century and was now growing back as a typical New England forested landscape—white pine and hemlock giving way to oak, maple, ash, and birch. There were a good-size vernal pool and two impressive rock formations—the Boulders, and Boulders Two. The woods were bounded on all sides by roads and houses, but inside they were quiet and deep.

I started wandering the woods to get away from adults, and because on those days after a visit to the hospital I had nothing else to do. I was forbidden to play sports. Doctor's orders. We had no television, and my brothers and sister where in school. And visits to the hospital left me in an agony of both fear and embarrassment. To start with, there was the problem of getting to the hospital in broad daylight on a day when everybody else was in school.

Even when escorted by my mother and walking at her side, I worried and magnified the incongruity and unnaturalness of my being out and about on a school day. Adults moved about their business, but there were no other kids on the streets. That policeman in his patrol car—he was looking over at us with what seemed casual interest as we waited for the light to change, but I could see otherwise. The policeman was thinking, "Why is that kid not in school?"

A car mechanic stood to wipe his hands on a towel and looked over our way as we entered the hospital grounds. Perhaps an adult would think that was just an appreciative look at my mother and a small smile from the mechanic, but I knew otherwise. You could easily see what he was thinking: "Boy that kid must be in real tough shape. 'Cardiac Clinics.' Only old people go there. A sad case."

Or later, after my surgery, Miss Z, my second-grade teacher (I had changed schools by then), calling me over during recess along with a bunch of boys that I had been galloping about with. "You are running too much. You're out of breath. I want you to stay here with me by the swings and not run for the rest of recess."

Later, incredulous questions from my friend Gary Yates and others. "Why did she make you stop running? What's the matter with you?"

I lied: "I hurt my ankle."

The truth was I had been born with a serious heart condition, a constricted pulmonary heart valve that left me short of breath, wheezing, and with intermittent chest pains. It had been that way since the day, sometime in my first year, when my mother took me to our family doctor for my first checkup.

Dr. Desautell, who had also delivered me, smiled and chatted with my mother while he placed his stethoscope on my chest. And then he stopped smiling, fell silent, and lifted his head from my chest. He frowned, shook his head slightly, and bent down to listen again. The second time he kept the stethoscope on my chest for a long time, moving it up and down and even around to my back.

My mother, a pretty woman of 28 with a husband just back from World War II and a growing family, held me and tried to remember if Dr. Desautell had been this thorough with her older boys. Dr. Desautell finished, looked over at my mother, started to say something, and then stopped. Abruptly, he put his stethoscope back to my chest. He listened for a third time, but quickly now. Then he removed his stethoscope, placed it carefully on the table, drew a deep breath, glanced at me, and then looked my mother in the eye. "Celia," he said, "Celia, there is something wrong with his ticker."

My mother didn't believe him. She dressed me quickly and rushed from the office in tears, sure that Dr. Desautell had made a mistake. She carried me around to other doctors for nearly a year, seeking a medical opinion that would contradict Dr. Desautell. She never found it.

The doctors in the local hospital in the Berkshires pondered over me for a long time after that, and for many visits, "This is a young man's future," they kept saying to my mother. "We need to do something." My parents finally agreed. I was removed from my classroom with Sister Agnes Marie, and one morning found myself riding to Boston in a big white station wagon of the American Heart Association.

We were poor, a family with six kids by then. We had no car. Mrs. Smith of the American Heart Association, Berkshire Chapter, concocted some business that needed doing in Boston and then offered to drive my mother and me to Children's Hospital. I had no idea why I was entering this big hospital in Boston.

There was a quiet nun in blue who talked to my mother and me in a small chapel. Later, there was an operating room, bright with large white lights overhead, and a nurse standing over me as I lay on my back, first offering a lollipop that I never got to unwrap and then pressing a gray rubbery mask over my face while telling me to count to ten, and still later I woke up groggy, my chest hurting and swathed in bandages, my mother bending over me.

There were lots of cards and gifts. That was good. There was a kaleidoscope that I shook and viewed a dozen times a minute, a book about Davy Crockett, a small green plastic travel toothbrush kit (a real prize since it showed that I was a sophisticated boy who had been places), and, best of all, a get-well card somebody had given me with a brand-new one dollar bill in it—more money than I had ever seen in my life. All these gifts and attention would make my brothers and sister jealous. But there was a downside.

First, there was the long wait to return home. My mother remembers the event one way: My father was in the sanatorium, recovering from tuberculosis. She was at home with six kids, no car, no money, and no babysitter when the time came to retrieve me from the hospital, 140 miles away. Unable to get anybody to watch her children, she couldn't get to Boston on the appointed day and came for me the next day.

I remember the story this way: I was standing by an elevator in Children's Hospital in Boston waiting for my mother. I was six years old. Each time the elevator stopped, I stepped forward to look for her among the crowd of nurses, doctors, and brightly dressed visitors who emerged. When the elevator departed, I watched the red indicator arrows in the wall panel and tracked its descent until it reached the ground floor, where a new batch of people would be getting on. In a short time, the elevator would be returning to my floor, and my mother would be on it, and I would be going home.

I watched and waited like this for most of the morning, my suitcase at my feet. Finally, a nurse came for me and took me by the hand and with her free hand picked up my suitcase. Together we went back to my hospital room. "One more night," the nurse told me. "Just one more night, and you'll be going home. Now how about an ice cream soda?" Where I came from that was an offer one never refuses.

I slurped my ice cream soda and wandered from my room, bored and restless. I tried the reception room where there are copies of *Look* and *Life* and other magazines scattered about on the gray plastic chairs. I glanced at the pictures in both magazines, but after a while I was bored and restless again. And I was worried. Why did my mother not come for me? I tried to remember, did she kiss me goodbye days ago after my surgery? Perhaps not. And what did that mean if she didn't? The nurse looked in on me, offered me another ice cream soda, which I accepted, and I asked the nurse for a pencil and paper.

And then I spent the rest of that long day drawing a map of my woods. They were large dark woods with hidden ponds, great pine trees, mossy swamps, shady lanes, and a sprawling sun-drenched field. I mapped it all out from memory and felt better.

At some point after the surgery, I began asking my mother and father about jobs for a boy with a heart condition. No, my father told me not unkindly, the FBI was out. Same with being a policeman or fireman. He said that you had to be a perfect specimen for those jobs. I pondered that as I walked my woods. By now there was a family dog that joined me. Skip, a large dark collie and shepherd mix, loved to charge through the woods, ranging in front and to the sides of me as I followed favorite trails to the Boulders, to Shady Lane, to Boulders Two, to the Old Pine Woods, and to Crane's Field (named for a prominent local family, not a bird).

Once, on a sun-streaked spring afternoon, several older boys found me in the woods. I had been poking about on the edge of Crane's Field when I saw them coming. They loomed over me, ominous and tough—not boys really—mostly teenagers, big guys with black engineer's boots, mounds of hair sculpted into place with Vaseline, cigarette packs tucked into rolled-up sleeves.

"What are you doing here?" somebody demanded.

Foolishly, I admitted the truth. "I'm counting rabbit holes in this field," I said, holding up my notebook as validation. "This is kind of my woods, and I thought I'd make a map of where the rabbits live."

"Counting rabbit holes," somebody sneered.

"What's that book?" somebody else asked, pointing at my *Golden Guide to Birds.*

"Well there are also these birds with a white chest and two big black bands on the chest. A whole flock of them; they come here every year. I'm counting them too."

Several of the older boys scowled menacingly. One reached down to grab my notebook. "What a creep," he said, and threw my notebook into a patch of tangled highbush blueberries. Another stepped up close, jabbed his finger an inch from my face, and then pointed up to the sky. "Look," he commanded. I looked up and the bad boy kicked my ankles with a swift scything stroke that sent me sprawling. Things were looking grim. But then one of the bad boys paused and looked down at me.

"Hey," he said to his companions, pointing a grease-stained index finger at me. "This looks like Denny Conuel's little brother."

His companions paused. One said, "Denny Conuel is the starting center on the football team."

"The football team sticks together," another bad boy said with the tone of one who has studied a complex subject deeply and come to some inalterable conclusions.

Clearly, the possibility that Denny would come looking for these young miscreants with half the Pittsfield High football team backing him up gave pause. Wisely, for once in my life, I kept my mouth shut.

Denny had quit the football team four days ago, but I wasn't telling.

The bad boys, however, were unaware of this. I said nothing to enlighten them. Finally one of them said. "Let him be. Who needs all the hassles?"

I have been back to those woods several times as an adult. The distance between the Boulders and Crane's Field has shrunk dramatically. The hike to Boulders Two, once a daunting trek not lightly undertaken, is now a twelve-minute walk along a well-tended path. The big deep pond that appeared every spring near Crane's Field has molded itself into damp wooded hollows and a shallow vernal pool with a few tadpoles. Crane's Field is still there, but I haven't seen the flocks of birds with white chests and dark breast bands (probably killdeer) that I used to spot—though I did see an indigo bunting on my last visit several years ago.

Eventually, the visits to the heart doctors ceased when I came home around age 12 from my first visit on my own and told my mother, "They just want to operate on me again, and I just want to be left alone."

Eventually, my rambles in the woods ceased too, replaced by a deep fondness for a 1957 Ford, two-tone blue, four-on-the-floor, wide whitewall tires, and a really decent radio that could pick up Joey Reynolds, the Emperor of the Nighttime, from faraway Buffalo.

But then many years later, in springtime, as a freshman at the University of Massachusetts in Amherst, I stood for the first time on the banks of the Connecticut River, New England's Great River, and it all came tumbling back.

I was on a field trip with a class of geology students inspecting the Triassic redbeds, one of the Connecticut River's distinctive rock formations. The geology teacher called out dates and rocks to the class, but his words were lost in the high wind that was whipping off the river. I stood there on the riverbank looking out across the blue-gray waters thinking what a small piece of time and landscape were captured here in this moment, and how this somehow brought me back to the woods where I had wandered as a boy.

I walked away from the group and stood on a ledge overlooking the water. It was just me and the river and nobody else, as it had been in the woods when I was a boy. I can capture this if I try hard enough, I thought. I'll write this all down. Standing there on the banks of the Connecticut, watching the river roll on to the sea, I flipped open my geology notebook, intended for scholarly observations, and started writing, hampered greatly by the high wind that tore at my pages.

I've been writing ever since. I write about the natural world because it is my excuse to go poking about in places and landscapes that have meant a lot to me—especially when I was a lost boy many years ago wandering on the frontiers of open-heart surgery. ❧

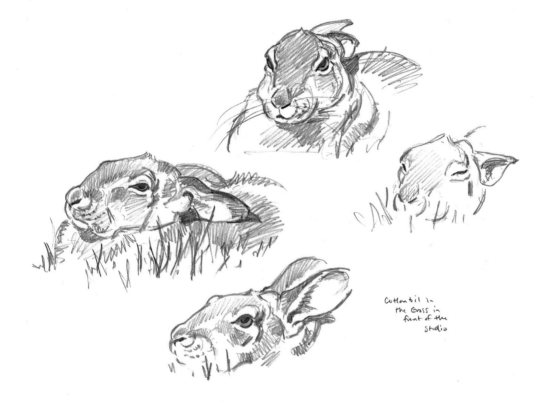

Cottontail in the Grass in front of the studio

SALVAGE

by Sarah Goodman

The world will go on,
and just
having been will be
enough.

The ducks will float in the marsh,
just like you told us, and I will want

to cross the water to them.
But I will stand, as you did,
with a lens and a longing, watching

ducks, dories, sandpipers
gather and disperse.

—for Miriam

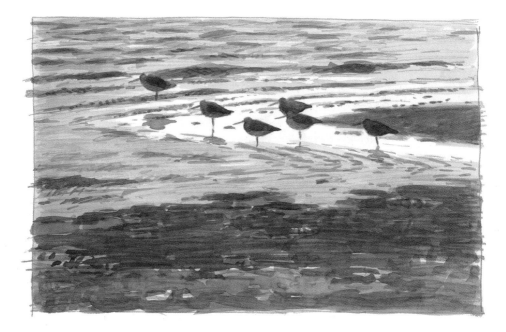

Saved by Swifts
by Richard Mabey

It's October, an Indian summer. I'm standing on the threshold like some callow teenager, about to move house for the first time in my life. I've spent more than half a century in this place, in this undistinguished, comfortable town house on the edge of Chiltern Hills, and had come to think we'd reached a pretty good accommodation. To have all mod cons on the doorstep of the quirkiest patch of countryside in south-east England had always seemed just the job for a rather solitary writing life. I'd use the house as a ground-base, and do my living in the woods, or in my head. I liked to persuade myself that the Chiltern landscape, with its folds and free-lines and constant sense of surprise, was what had shaped my prose, and maybe me too. But now I am upping sticks and fleeing to the flatlands of East Anglia.

My past, or lack of it, had caught up with me. I'd been bogged down in the same place for too long, trapped by habits and memories. I was clotted with rootedness. And in the end I'd fallen ill and run out of words. My Irish grandfather, a day-worker who rarely stayed in one house long enough to pay the rent, knew what to do at times like this. In that word that catches all the shades of escape, from the young bird's flutter from the nest to the dodging of someone in trouble, he'd flit.

Yet hovering on the brink of this belated initiation, all I can do is think back again, to another wrenching journey. It had been a few summers before, when I was just beginning to slide into a state of melancholy and senselessness that were incomprehensible to me. I was due to go for a holiday in the Cévennes with some old friends, a few weeks in the limestone *causses* that had become something of a tradition, but could barely summon up enough spirit to leave home. Somehow I made it, and the Cévennes were, for that brief respite, as healing as ever, a time of sun and hedonism and companionship.

But towards the end of my stay something happened which lodged in my mind like a primal memory: a glimpse of another species' rite of passage. I'd travelled south to the Herault for a couple of days, and stayed overnight with my friends in a crooked stone house in Octon. In the morning we came across a fledgling swift beached in the attic. It had fallen out of nest and lay with its crescent wings stretched out stiffly, unable to take off. Close to, its juvenile plumage wasn't the enigmatic black of those careering midsummer silhouettes, but a marbled mix of charcoal-grey and brown and powder-white. And we could see the price it paid for being so exquisitely adapted to life that would be spent almost entirely in the air. Its prehensile claws, four facing to the front, were mounted on little more than feathered stumps, half-way down its body. We picked it up, carried it to the window and hurled it out. It was just six weeks old, and having its maiden flight and first experience of another species all in the same moment.

But whatever its emotions, they were overtaken by instinct and natural bravura. It went into a downward slide, winnowing furiously, skimmed so close to the road that we all gasped, and then flew up strongly towards the south-east. It would not touch down again until it came back to breed in two summers' time. How many miles is that? How many wing-beats? How much time off?

I tried to imagine the journey that lay ahead of it, the immense odyssey along a path never flown before, across chronic war-zones and banks of Mediterranean gunmen, through precipitous changes of weather and landscape. Its parents and siblings had almost certainly left already. It would be flying the 6,000 miles entirely on its own, on a course mapped out—or at least sketched out—deep in its central nervous system. Every one of its senses would be helping to guide it, checking its progress against genetic memories, generating who knows what astonishing experiences of consciousness. Maybe, like many seabirds, it would be picking up subtle changes in air-borne particles as it passed over seas and aromatic shrubland and the dusty thermals above African townships. It might be riding a magnetic trail detected by iron-rich cells in its forebrain. It would almost certainly be using, as navigation aids, landmarks whose shapes fitted templates in its genetic memories, and the sun too, and, on clear nights, the big constellations—which, half-way through its journey, would be replaced by a quite different set in the night sky of the southern hemisphere. Then, after three or four weeks, it would arrive in South Africa and earn its reward of nine months of unadulterated, aimless flying and playing. Come the following May, it and all the other first-year birds would come back to Europe and race recklessly about the sky just for the hell of it. That is what swifts do. It is their ancestral, unvarying destiny for the non-breeding months. But you would need to have a very sophisticated view of pleasure to believe they also weren't also 'enjoying' themselves.

When that May came round I was blind to the swifts for the first time in my life. While they were *en fête* I was lying on my bed with my face away from the window, not really caring if I saw them again or not. In a strange and ironic turn-about, I had become the incomprehensible creature adrift in some insubstantial medium, out of kilter with the rest of creation. It didn't occur to me at the time, but maybe that is the way our whole species is moving....

So I'm thinking again about my feelings for that beached, fledgling swift. Where did they come from? I don't eat swifts, or aspire to have them as pets. I don't feel they need my protection, having existed perfectly independently on the planet for millions of years. And in a view of the world based on 'resource conservation', swifts are almost certainly irrelevant. They are not (yet) endangered. No important predator depends on them (and if it did, we would then have to ask what use that is). The planet's linked ecosystems—what James Lovelock has christened Gaia—would give no more than a sigh if they vanished. It would be testing credulity to suggest that one day they might be the source of a drug against, say, air-sickness, distilled from their prodigious balancing organs; or that their scrabbled-together nests (made from flotsam gathered from the air) could provide the inspiration for low-cost building designs. No, swifts do not pass the critical tests of endangerment or usefulness.

Yet they touch and connect with us in deep and subtle ways. We do not know what it would be like to live through a summer without them. They are part of our myths of spring and the South, a crucial element in that great gift to the temperate zone, the migration and settlement of summer birds. 'An annual barter of 'food for light', Aldo Leopold wrote of migration in America, in which 'the whole continent receives as net profit a wild poem dropped from the murky skies.' They are the most pure expression of flight, an ability which is still remembered somewhere deep in our nervous system. Swifts have become, I think, our twenty-first-century equivalent of the Romantics' nightingales— cryptic, rhapsodic, electrifying—but happy to be all these things at high speed in the middle of an urban landscape. Like the nightingale's 'darkling' song, the swift's black silhouette and utterly aerial existence give them a pliability of meaning.

When I was at school I longed so much for their return that I used to walk about on May Day clutching my blazer collar for luck. Later, when I was about seventeen, they became romantic emblems of high summer. I sang in early music choir in those days, and on June evenings we rehearsed in a local parish church with the local girls' school perched on the opposite side of the chancel. The swifts screamed round the tower, and past the stained-glass windows lit by the low sun—a shrill descant to our own warblings. It was a haunting scene of unrequited courtly lust, and though swifts are now beyond the range of my hearing, I can still recall the sound of those evenings, along with the forbidden thrill of the girls' green gingham dresses.

In my adult life swifts have become more mysterious, not a symbol of anything in particular, but creatures made of the same cells and tissues as me yet living on another, almost unknowable plane. Their existence in—and sometimes, it seems, on—air is more cryptic than the livelihood which myriads of creatures make suspended in and supported by water. Swifts eat, sleep and mate on the wing. They gather windblown debris for nests and bathe in the rain ('they take showers', wrote William Fiennes). All over Europe—in that extraordinary town of birds, Trujillo, and lost on a motorway somewhere just outside Montpellier—I've stood mesmerised as they hurtled past me at waist level, wondering what they made of me. Were they aware that—earthbound and ponderous—I was even alive?

Mostly I used to watch swifts down by the canal in my old home in the

Chilterns. I'd go to a pub an hour or two before sunset, and lose myself in their vespers ritual. They nested, a dozen or so pairs, in the eaves of a row of Victorian terraced houses, and in a disused factory that used to manufacture insecticides. And on warm, still evenings the young neighbourhood singletons would form a loose flock, trawling insects a couple of hundred feet above the town centre. They looked as if they were milling about haphazardly, like ash specks over a bonfire, but would cross and swoop over each other's paths without missing a wing-beat.

Then some ancient compulsion took over, quite pointless unless you are prepared to grant birds a sense of pure physical relish in their power of flight. At the edges of the swarm the birds began to wheel, wings stiff. One by one they dived down to a lower altitude, and began to fly and chase, first in pairs then in accumulating strands, until maybe thirty birds were careering together in a mass. They became a ragged black comet, fizzing with activity as birds throttled back, feathered, did spectacular left-right wing-tilts to avoid collisions. The comet hurtled between the factory buildings, calling to the sitting birds inside, banked like a gang of motorcyclists to take the curve back over the new wharfside flats. They seemed to be following tracks in the air that only they could see—but would then spectacularly run off them. They'd disappear only to somehow reappear behind me. Then abruptly, at no visible signal, they would fling apart and fly off leisurely in different directions, making for the high air again.

I never saw the actual moment when they disappeared for rest. I suspect they gained altitude rather like an aircraft, flying out of the town on a gradual gradient. But I have seen a film of the image south-east England's sleep-bound swifts make on air-traffic-control radar. As darkness falls all the aircraft on the screen are obliterated by an ethereal halo of bright coalescing spots, each one an individual group of swifts, bound for that state of total otherness—invisible, aerial slumber.

Witness Tree

by Sophie Wadsworth

Phil and his wife Beth prune, feed and worry
but refuse to cut. Wide as a barn door,
the sycamore is older than anything
in sight, and we pray it will outlive us.
We stand in rain, talking about rain
and what men do to each other.
The branches turn slick and rain
flows in sepia streaks down the trunk.

Also called buttonwood, this one is known
as The Whipping Tree. Here in 1783, a Shaker
named Abijah Worster was bound and lashed
by a mob until a General rode by
and set the man free, telling the crowd
to whip him instead.

For a talisman, I pocket downy fruit,
packed with gold-brown seeds.
Our soldiers come home without their limbs—
and we send new ones overseas.
We could do worse than planting sycamores
whose shade we do not expect to see.
Where plates of bark have fallen away,
the pale green cambium shines—
by the inch, the heartwood keeps growing.
One limb now spans the road, its branches reaching.

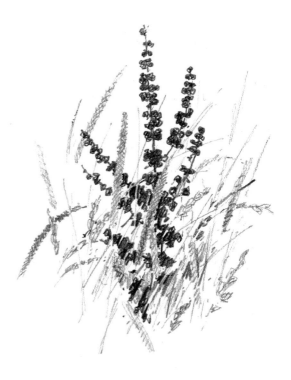

Solace and the Art of Scything
by John Hanson Mitchell

It's seven o'clock in the morning on June ninth and birdsong and sun are all abroad in the land. I'm sitting on my porch, drinking coffee and eyeing the grasses in a sweep of greensward that runs from the front of my house down a slope to a little shady alcove of clipped hemlocks on the eastern side of the property. My intention today, if things go well, is to mow the grasses, wildflowers, and ground covers that make up the body of the plant material in this expanse of open space. In order to accomplish this task, I'll use a scythe, a tool that was perfected sometime in the twelfth century and whose basic structure has remained unchanged ever since.

Cutting this section of what my old mother used to call "my grounds" is not a major piece of work; I could probably cut the whole strip in fifteen minutes or so with a ride-on power mower. But I prefer to make a project of it and mow by hand, mainly so that I can enjoy the morning. And it's a beautiful day withal; the little pine warblers are stitching the trees together with their sewing machine song; the cardinals are whistling in the thickets on the south side of the property; the indigo buntings are singing; the dew is on the vine; and (as far as I know) all's right with the world.

In point of fact, all's wrong with the world. Earlier that year, a huge international coalition of Christian armies had once again invaded the Levant and local forces had, as expected, risen up to defend themselves. There was fighting in the mountains to the east; fighter planes and Howitzers shelled ancient villages where, over the centuries, the local people, of necessity, would cast their lots with whichever violent tribal warlord held sway. To the southwest, the deserts were burning; the rivers were fouled with the wastes of war, the great marshes at the confluence of the two great rivers east of the Fertile Crescent were drained, and the Ma'dan, a generally nonviolent unaligned tribe of swamp dwellers, were either killed or evicted.

But all that is out there. Not here in the garden. Not this morning, at least. And anyway, in the long run, what can those of us who attempt to live quiet lives without praise or blame possibly do about an international conflict undertaken by distant heads of states over questionable issues about which we have very little influence.

With this in mind, I shoulder my scythe and walk around to the top of the greensward and begin to cut.

It rained last night. The clovers and grasses are wet and heavy, and the sun is glinting in little sparkling lights on the leaves of the ajugas and violets—perfect conditions for scything. The scythe snatches low, and the grasses fall easily as I begin to mow along the first row. I can hear the swish of the blade, the chatter of the wrens, and the chuck of the local robins, and smell the rich odor of cut grass and pungent weeds.

Scything is notoriously hard work if you go at it with brute force, but easy, even pleasurable and contemplative work, if you take your time, and rest periodically to smell the earth and listen to the birds and the crickets.

This is the first cutting, which is always the smoothest and freshest. I take a few swipes and walk on, take another swing and another step, and move on, slowly sweeping and cutting, sweeping and cutting, and mowing eastward down

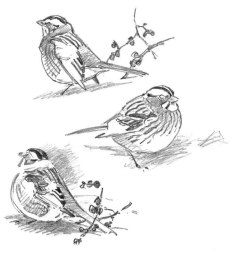

the line, leaving a two- or three-foot swathe of fallen grasses in my wake. The moist scent of fresh herbage rises around me, the birds sing in apparent unison, and from the farm on the other side of the hill I can hear a dog barking lazily.

It's easy to forget that elsewhere things are falling apart—wars raging in the Middle East, wars in Sub-Saharan Africa, civil unrest in Middle Europe, crime in the streets at home, corruption in governments, vast gulfs between the rich and the poor, armed madmen loosed on the towns. It's all storm and chaos and noise.

But not here.

In his novella, *Candide*, Voltaire may have summed up the state in which I currently find myself. Having traveled the world with his various companions, and having seen all manner of disasters, including the deadly Lisbon earthquake and the local Inquisition, and having retreated finally to a small farm in Turkey, Candide announces that in the face of it all there's nothing to be done but cultivate your garden.

In some ways that was the original purpose of a cultivated ornamental garden. It was a hedge against reality. The creators of the great Italian villa gardens of the Renaissance were well aware of this fact. Streets and alleyways were plague ridden and squalid in those chaotic decades; footpads and highwaymen, and warring city-state armies rattled through the countryside and the clamor of war was in the air. Better to stay in the walled villa gardens, lounging by the wellhead among the quinces and the ilex hedges.

I learned to cut with a scythe shortly after I moved to this land. I had recently been in the Azores, in the interior of the island of São Miguel, and saw an old man cutting a smooth green lawn with a scythe. I knew that the traditional American yeoman used a scythe to cut hay and wheat. But I had never seen anybody mow a lawn with one. In my broken, schoolboy Portuguese, I fell into conversation with the old man and he let me try to mow. The trick, I learned, was to keep the blade very sharp and cut low and slow. Actually, I never did learn the real art. But I still like to pretend.

No more than twenty yards into my work that morning, in midswing, I saw something leap in an angled arc out for the jeweled grass tangle—a wood frog. This is a good garden for frogs. In the forest just northwest of the property, there are two vernal pools where wood frogs breed, and, since this is hardly a manicured, pesticide-laden, neatly mown piece of land, they take refuge here. I can understand this. I'm doing the same thing. Theirs is a dangerous world, so dangerous that—unlike my own species—they are approaching the endangered species list. They eschew shorn lawns, paved driveways, and parking lots, none of which they will find here. But their presence in the long grasses is actually a problem for me.

Scything is quiet work, save for the whisper of the cutting blade. Frogs, snakes, grasshoppers, crickets, toads, and spiders (and also on a couple of occasions baby bunnies) do not hear the approaching scyther. This creates a dilemma. If ever I mow this swathe with a power mower, which I do every couple of years just to make a fresh start, long before the machine comes their way, the local denizens flee to safety. I hate to confess that more than once I have speared a toad by this scything work. Even the memory is unpleasant, and sometimes gets me wondering whether I should just let the whole garden go wild and stop cutting and trimming and planting.

In fact, perhaps cutting and pruning could be considered by some ethicists as a form of plant cruelty. A clipped grass blade or tree branch is in some ways a brutal injury to the organism. Plants have evolved the ability to grow back, but would it not be better to let them grow freely as they would in wild nature? I actually posed this question once to a biologist with a decidedly ethical bent and she assured me that it's okay to cut grass; it will grow back with vigor. "It's what plants do," she said.

In any case, the fact is if I quit managing this land the whole place would be taken over by invasive plants in a matter of years. As it is there is a lot of diversity on my grounds. I did a rough survey of the plants and animals in this acre-and-a-half garden one year and counted well over 2,000 species, which, I was told by an ecologist, is probably a very conservative count.

No matter, whether wild or tamed, the modern world is dangerous for wildlife: speeding cars, unchecked development everywhere, pesticides, climate change. It's also dangerous for people. A few weeks ago, just about the time that the violets, ajugas, clovers, and Quaker ladies were abloom in the mead, a mad man with a shaved head and an AKA-40 wandered into a public event and started randomly shooting people. The police stopped him. But as if to finish the business, another disturbed individual began shooting up the streets in front of a mosque. More shootings, this time in Texas. Police killed an unarmed man in Florida. There were riots. Somebody tried to break into the White House. A friend of mine got mugged not far from the Boston Common, and everywhere there was bedlam.

When I first came to this property, I started using the scythe to mow the blackberry brambles and rampant orchard grasses that grew just outside the backdoor of the farmhouse where I lived. It was all part of a little fantasy I was playing out at the time. The place was a wreck in those early years—an early nineteenth-century farmhouse with canted walls, a caved-in barn, a few old apple trees, poison ivy everywhere, and on a rise behind the house, where a former apple orchard once grew, a block of ominous white pines that seemed to absorb all surrounding light.

My idea was to fix the place up and grow things there. Restore the land in other words. But I wanted to do it in the old way. Hand-tools only. It took me years, but slowly, working with the scythe, a mattock, shovels, and rakes, I managed to clear enough land to create a semblance of a pseudo-Italianate garden, a landscape design I had come to appreciate over the years. By the time I finally finished, I was living in a different house on the property, a house based on the designs of the mid-nineteenth-century landscape architect and house designer Andrew Jackson Downing.

Downing was a member of a loosely organized group of gardeners and landscapers known as the Genteel Romantics who favored integrated pleasure grounds complete with woodland groves mixed with ornamental gardens, fruiting orchards, and waterworks. Essentially they were escapists. They were contemporaries of Thoreau, Emerson, and the Abolitionists, but they chose to pretend that nothing was wrong with the world. They loved nature, but they believed in living modulated orderly lives. They weren't radical, nor were they Transcendentalists; they sought only the peace of nature.

I appreciate their philosophy, but I'm not that good at pretending. I try though. Anyway, I'm not the only one who has tried to escape into the myth of the garden in order to survive in the face of the absurdity of war, the destruction of the environment, the violence of the streets, and all the other ills wrought by the successful primate species known as Cro-Magnon. The garden is indeed a sanctuary if you can willingly suspend disbelief while working there. It can even be a sacred place for those who believe in that sort of thing. I used to know an older gardener years ago, an irreligious man, who somewhat ironically given his religious nonbeliefs used to talk about "cathedral time," by which he meant the hours he spent in his garden.

Halfway down the line I've planted a little circular garden bed in the center of the swath with an ornate urn, planted with long-lived annuals—yet another Italianate flourish in this American garden, and also a good refuge for snowy tree crickets. Later in the summer, I can always hear them repeating their interminable birdlike chirps in this spot, a sultry languorous sound that always seems to me to speak of fecundity and primordial life. I believe it was Nathaniel Hawthorne who wrote somewhere that, if you could hear moonlight, it would sound like a snowy tree cricket.

As early as late April you can hear meadow crickets calling from the grassy thickets here, also field crickets, and then in late June the fireflies collect in the air above this section of the garden. After that, in August, the snowy tree crickets, and then the katydids, begin calling from the surrounding treetops, and then the dragonflies arrive. All this is made possible by the fact that the scythe, in spite of my best efforts, does not leave behind a shorn lawn. Even after I've cut and raked up the grasses, the vegetation is high enough to shelter all these native species of insects. This section of the garden, and in fact all the open areas, is more like medieval mead, a mix of grasses, herbs, and forbs. From April to mid-November there is always a variety of color here because of the mix of plant material.

I sweep on, one swing, step, another swing, step, little by little the land is transformed.

In some ways I hate cutting down this mixed tangle of grasses and wildflowers. But the fact is, I know that if I let it go the grasses and flowering plants will go to seed, turn brown, and lose their vitality. The crickets and the sparrows wouldn't care. In fact they would probably prosper on the seeds and the shelter. But I like the flowers and the new grown fresh greenery.

Out on the main road, about a quarter of a mile south of this property, I hear the wail of a siren, soon joined by the yelp of police cars. Something unfortunate has happened. Violence on the roads perhaps.

There's no visual disturbance here in the garden; I can't see anything but trees and greenery from this land. Noise is the only intruder. That and the daily news. I hate reading the news nowadays, but I do it anyway. Last week there was a major conflict in the ongoing desert war just east of the ancient city of Uruk. A big tank battle. Many casualties on both sides. This was not a good year for world peace.

Farther south, in Sub-Saharan Africa, powerful tribes had clashed, citing ancient grievances. A victorious army clipped through the jungle terrain with the same ferocity as the warring armies in the north and east. Villages were attacked and burned, and an immense number of refugees fled eastward and southward, moving unseen through the vast Ituri Forest in central Africa, living on bush meat and thereby threatening the existence of local, and in some cases endangered, species of forest animals. The pursuing army cut a swath of destruction through the forest, driving the peaceful Mbuti Pygmies deeper and deeper into their forest sanctuary.

There is nothing new as far as the disasters of war are concerned. Save for a period of universal peace in northern India under the reign of King Ashoka around 323 BC, and a curious 100-year period of religious tolerance and general peace during the Caliphate of Cordoba in tenth-century Spain, the world has been characterized by violence.

If I have my histories right, the scythe as we know it was invented around the time of the First Crusade when a vast international force of Christian armies, encouraged by the religious fanatic Peter the Hermit, fought their way down through the Italian peninsula and on to Antioch, Byzantium, and the Near East and finally, after two years of warring, to Jerusalem. There were many subsequent Crusades, ten in all, and there were many wars in the region before that and many afterward, one of which was currently in progress on that June morning. Earlier in that month there was a pitched tank battle not far from the Via Maris, a place that archeologists discovered a few years ago, evidence of what may have been the first organized war involving armies and sieges and the spread of empire—the city of Uruk, in this case.

We seem to have to live with this as a species. No one has yet beaten swords into ploughshares, even after generations of prophets and antiwar efforts and religions crying out for peace and love.

One day in the early years on this property, I was scything in the lower reaches of the mead nearer to the road when someone called up to me from the street.

"Cutting in the old way," he shouted, in a lilting Swedish accent.

I knew the voice; it was Sven, an acquaintance of mine who I used to chat up whenever I saw him walking by. Sven was a man out of an older Europe. Sweden along with Switzerland is one of the few European countries that has managed to remain neutral in the course of disastrous modern wars. Sven had a way of dismissively turning his head sideways and clucking whenever we mentioned the calamity of the news, as if to say: whatever can we do? Even though he was in his eighties when I knew him, he used to hike the mile and a half to town and back. Sometimes on return, he would take a shortcut and pass through the woods east of the house to collect firewood. I'd see him making his way up the road, carrying heavy logs on his shoulder for his stove. He was one of three or four old farmers who had been working the land in these parts since the 1920s, when a new wave of immigrant farmers replaced the original Yankee owners.

Sven and I chatted about scything for a while, how he and his father and brothers and cousins used to cut the meadows back in Sweden and how the adults would use the occasion to celebrate. They'd sing while they mowed and sometimes would hold a ring dance when the hay was in and get drunk and carry on late into the purple midsummer night.

Sven got me thinking about the famous scything scene from *Anna Karenina* in which the egalitarian conflicted estate owner, Levin, spends the day out in the fields with his peasants, trying to keep up with them as they cut the rows of wheat. He falls behind, totally fatigued, while they continue on with their slow rhythmic swings. But as he enters into the pace of the work, he slips into a state of unconsciousness, as if the scythe alone is doing the work. In short, he reaches that condition of timeless bliss offered by those who meditate regularly. He does not recognize the passage of hours until someone calls out to him that it is dinnertime.

It occurred to me later that I was a little like Levin, in an American sort of way (although hardly as rich). Scything calms the mind. The ambience of nature obliterates the world beyond the moment; you live in the reality of the rhythmic work, the sweep of muscle, the unity of earth and air.

I grew up in an old suburb outside of New York City, and although I had farmers and watermen in my family of origin from the Eastern Shore of Maryland and had even milked a few cows in my time, I was essentially a city boy, not a countryman. Now, like Levin, I had retreated to the countryside to play the yeoman. I am sure my local farming confidants found me mildly amusing.

But never mind. All this is good for you. Recent peer-reviewed studies have determined that exposure to green space is salutary. So of course is exercise. So is meditation, and the therapy of certain aromas, as of fresh-cut grass, and even the presence of organic compounds known as phytoncides that are released by forest trees and shrubs. Also exposure to the sun—in spite of the possible danger of skin cancer. It's the best source of vitamin D, as well as regulating melatonin levels, which contribute to healthful sleep patterns and thus have a positive effect on mood.

I continue to mow eastward toward the shady hemlock arbor and the road, slowly cutting south to north, north to south, and back again, and all the while laying down the thatch of long grasses behind me. Whenever I stop to rest, I look back at my handiwork and notice that the tapestry of fallen grasses is alive with small insects, crawling, leaping, and burrowing back down into the tangle, their world temporarily upset, but unharmed. They will carry on; the grasses and flowers will grow back and life will go on. At least until winter.

At the garden bench in the hemlock alcove I lean the scythe against a tree and sit down for a spell. I've made four circuits of this little patch so far, and there is a great oblong stand of uncut grass and clover in the middle of the space. Not much more to cut.

I give the scythe a few licks with the whetstone and then start down the island of remaining grasses, cutting and sweeping.

I asked old Sven once to show me how they cut hay back in the old country. He took up the scythe, went to the middle of the meadow, and began to cut from the inside out, making ever-widening concentric circles. Another old boy I knew, who used to cut salt hay with a scythe on the North River marshes when he was young, told me to cut from the outside in. Levin and his peasants, as I recall, worked down long rows, side by side in an angled line. In my little plot, I go along the edges first and work inward. I notice that later in the season, when the frogs and the snakes are out and about, they tend to move inward to the uncut swathe. So before I cut the final stand, I walk in and literally kick them out before I cut down their last refuge.

The sun is drifting across the forest canopy on the other side of the road at this point. The morning birdsong has diminished to a few errant calls from the catbirds and the ever-present house wrens. Summer is coming in; the mead is cut; and I'm getting hungry.

One more pass and I'll be done.

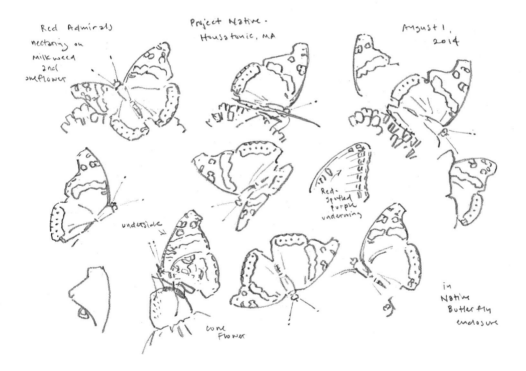

Red Admirals nectaring on Milkweed and suflower

Project Native. Houssatonic, MA

August 1, 2014

underside

Red-Spotted Purple underwing

coneFlower

in Native Butterfly enclosure

Visitation

by Christopher Locke

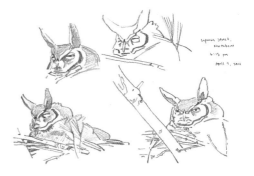

Not the boot-sucking clam bed,
Sophie stuck up to her knees, tide out and rocks
gulping at their own nakedness.

Not the trails scraped in snowmelt
winding the nearby woods where she lost
one of her mittens as we spied deer prints
and dog prints thinned to crystal relics.

Not the quick
slip to pavement, leg rubied in small
scratches, lower lip quivering, incapable
of holding so many indignities in such short
order. No. It was Sophie uttering her desire,
limping now, to just once see an owl's face
"…in real life," until all of us stopped dumb
in our tracks on that wet country road
as one appeared, barred and mute
in the twilit branches above. We stared

a good, long time until *I* hooted, and the owl
lifted away into its deeper silence.

And there was Sophie,
shy again, walking upright, even as we returned
to the house where all the windows were dark.

—*for Sophie, age 8*

Children of the Wired World
The Serious Threat to Human Contact with the Natural World that Comes in the Form of a Screen
by Michael J. Caduto

The sky watches us and listens to us. It talks to us, and it hopes we are ready to talk back…. Our God is the sky, and lives wherever the sky is. Our God is the sun and the moon, too; and our God is the people, if we remember to stay here. This is where we're supposed to be, and if we leave we lose God.

—10-year-old Hopi child, New Mexico

The World Health Organization defines health as "a state of complete physical, mental, and social well-being and not merely the absence of disease or infirmity." The word comes from the Old English *haelth*, being whole, well, or sound, and from the Old Norse *helge*, for holy or sacred. In practice, Western medicine has tended to view health as the science of preventing and curing disease. But a more holistic view, and one more in keeping with the origin of the word, is that health is a state of balance, an equilibrium that an individual has established with his or her social and physical environment.

In many indigenous cultures, the idea that health is rooted in a life lived in balance takes on an even deeper dimension: individual health is closely intertwined with family and community life, with cultural traditions, the natural world, and the spiritual realm. True health is inclusive of body, mind, and spirit.

When I was a child, my place of healing was a rocky outcrop called Billy Goat Bluff that overlooked the overgrown pasture of an old farm. There I sat for long stretches of time during periods of joy, stress, or pain, gathering myself in. Away from home or school, I had the world to myself—just the wind through the trees and the occasional bird flying by. No one could see me or touch me. I could sing at the top of my voice and no one heard. In later years, when I was in my teens, no matter how unpredictable and mercurial life seemed, Billy Goat Bluff remained a touchstone to my center of gravity. Nature became my best friend because she was a constant green polestar—always there when I needed her.

We now understand more clearly and scientifically how nature benefits children physically, emotionally, and psychologically as well as intellectually and spiritually. From the need for children to understand where their food comes from to the profound impacts of climate change throughout the world, there is a clear relationship between the state of nature and its impact on youth. Research has consistently shown that playing in green areas promotes creativity and critical-thinking skills. Educational programs that engage children in extended outdoor learning experiences have been found to generate positive outgrowths such as a greater ability to pay attention and achieve in reading, math, and social studies. Exposure to green spaces reduces stress, improves discipline, and enhances the ability to relate well and get along with others. Outdoor experiences even benefit eyesight and reduce the likelihood that a child will develop myopia.

And if all of this weren't enough, children are also *happier* when they get to spend time outdoors. Their lives are enriched and curiosity is piqued by the infinite variety of things to see and do among the plants and animals; the rocks, water, and sky. Anyone who has watched a group of children run out of a schoolhouse door during recess and fly across the playground, squealing with delight, knows how nature and play and happiness are all intertwined.

There may be risks when playing in the outdoors, everything from cuts and scrapes to broken bones, but long-term health problems that arise from spending thousands of sedentary hours indoors seated in front of a computer screen or other electronic device are far worse—impaired brain development, obesity, and even cardiovascular disease.

In the 1960s, when my friends and I were growing up with much of our time spent outdoors, whenever we got a cut or scrape we wore it to school like a badge of honor, proving we had the moxie to get hurt and come back to play another day. Today, as in the past, traditional peoples who live close to nature benefit from the experience of contact with their environments. The ancient stewardship practices that have enabled indigenous peoples to live sustainably with their world are woven into the fabric of their social, cultural, and spiritual lives; these traditions are also deeply rooted in practicality. Take care of your environment and people survive and live well; destroy your environment and everyone suffers. As American ecologist Aldo Leopold stated: "A thing is right when it tends to preserve the integrity, stability and beauty of the biotic community. It is wrong when it tends to do otherwise."

Developing a relationship with the natural world lays the foundation for raising children who will value and protect the health and well-being of the environment. Simply exposing children to nature for an extended period of time is an essential part of forming that bond. "If a child is to keep alive his inborn sense of wonder, he needs the companionship of at least one adult who can share it, rediscovering with him the joy, excitement, and mystery of the world we live in," wrote biologist Rachel Carson in her book *The Sense of Wonder*. We are all children of nature. Our sense of place is founded on many aspects of how we relate to the world around us.

Befriending the environment during the formative years, and experiencing the innate sense of communion between self and the natural world, have often become the inspiration and impetus for preserving the local landscape. Spurred on by a youthful passion and deep caring for nature, many environmental activists, educators, and authors were compelled to fight for their local environment at an early age when an outside agent of change, such as pollution or development, posed an immediate threat.

In our time, however, these former associations with nature are seriously threatened. Just a generation ago, no one could foresee a time when such a crisis would come. Children who had access to the outdoors spent most of their time swimming in ponds, catching turtles, and inventing imaginary worlds where trolls and fairies cavorted among frogs and dragonflies. In his book *Last Child in the Woods*, Richard Louv notes a University of Maryland study with findings that in 2013 half as many children in the United States ages 9 to 12 were spending time engaged in outdoor activities (fishing, hiking, gardening, going to the beach) than just six years earlier. This is the trend all around the world, in both urban and rural settings, and it's become endemic to children's experiences in modern society.

Nowadays, due to concerns over safety, highly structured schedules, and extreme focus on academic achievement from a very early age, reaching even into the pre-K years, children have very little open, unstructured, outdoor time to themselves, and far less control over their own free time. Furthermore, even as toddlers they turn to spending time on computers, cell phones, iPods, tablets, and myriad other electronic devices.

From Europe to the Middle East, from North America to Asia, research has proven that children are more connected to the content of their apps than they are to their surroundings. Whereas parents of earlier generations were eager to send their children outdoors—they were glad to have us out of their hair in fact and perfectly happy to leave us to our own wanderings—we now have a generation of parents who worry about the amount of time children spend with their electronic devices, and the accompanying health ramifications.

Not only do electronic devices separate children from nature, but their overuse has serious negative health impacts that are widespread and dangerous. According to a variety of recent studies, children using cell phones are less aware of their surroundings and are three times as likely to be killed or seriously injured in a traffic accident while walking to school. Overexposure to devices during a child's first two years, when the brain triples in size, can lead to impaired learning and delayed cognitive development. Youngsters who frequently look at screens can become impulsive, less disciplined, and prone to tantrums. Children who are allowed to have an electronic device in their bedroom run a 30 percent greater risk of being overweight. They also may experience sleeplessness and poor academic performance. Excessive screen time can increase the risk of depression, anxiety, and other forms of psychological malaise. Not to mention that the Internet can be addictive.

A study by the group Common Sense Media found that 17 percent of children who are 8 and younger use mobile devices every day; this number has more than doubled since 2011.

Research conducted by the American Academy of Pediatics (AAP) found that children today use some form of electronic entertainment seven hours each day on average. That amounts to 2,500 hours per year, equivalent to nearly three and a half months of 24-hour days each year.

In January 2015, Taiwan passed a law banning the use of electronic devices (iPads, TVs, and smartphones) by children under 2 years old. Parents who violate this law can be fined up to $1,500. The AAP and the Environmental Health Trust have issued recommendations for limitations on the use of devices by children, which include texting, watching TV, and using social media and the Internet. They recommend that families prohibit children under 2 years of age from TV and the Internet, and allowing no more than two hours of screen time per day for children over 2. They also suggest eliminating the use of electronic devices after bedtime and during mealtimes and keeping TVs and devices with Internet access out of children's rooms.

In order to live a healthy life, children need to find their center—that inner place where body, mind, and spirit are one—a core identity that is uniquely theirs and makes them who they are. How does a child accomplish this when he/she is bombarded by messages delivered through electronic media for seven hours each day—messages that are designed to manipulate that child to do or buy something, or to be persuaded toward a particular way of thinking or acting? Research shows that children gradually develop their second-order reasoning, or Theory of Mind— the ability to think for oneself and distinguish between one's own state of mind (knowledge, beliefs, desires, and intentions) and those of others.

Because it takes time for each child to develop a "mind of one's own," it clearly is not in the interest of fostering a child's mental, physical, and emotional health to expose that child to endless hours of propaganda. This is especially true for children under the age of 10. Even when children have developed their abilities for higher level, second-order reasoning, they need to be taught the skills necessary for examining what is behind the messages they are constantly experiencing.

In this way, they will be able to distinguish between what is healthy and what is not, and make their own critical decisions about what they want to accept or reject. With this awareness and these skills, youth can learn how to interact online in a way that is healthy and proactive rather than submissive and reactive.

With so many children displaced from the natural world because they spend much of their time immersed in the virtual world, some critical questions arise: How can we encourage children to engage with their real surroundings and develop a relationship with nature? How can we help their experience of nature to become the basis for a healthy life? Does the use of devices have any legitimate role in environmental education?

Some educators argue that electronic devices should play no role in environmental education because overexposure to the virtual world causes a serious disconnect between children and the real world they live in, including their social interactions and relationship to nature. By contrast, some suggest that electronic devices can be used to reach children in the virtual world through specially designed apps and online programs that teach about nature and encourage youth to go outside and experience the natural world for themselves. This is a subject of ongoing debate.

While the prevalence of devices presents daunting challenges, even children who were raised in an era when they spent much of their time playing outdoors, and had a healthier childhood, did not automatically grow up to become environmental stewards, nor did they necessarily understand the connection between a healthy environment and human health.

Most environmental education programs focus on increasing children's experiences, knowledge, and skills. Yet these critical building blocks of an environmental consciousness need to be laid upon a foundation of wisdom—the beliefs, values, and attitudes that can lead to a lifetime of environmental stewardship.

How do we bring stewardship down to earth for children? How can we weave care for earth into the warp and weft of a child's inner life? Every child lives a unique story that unfolds within the context of family and the greater narratives of culture. Help a child to actively create the story of a life well lived and you literally offer that child the gift of a lifetime and help each child to see how the story of his/her own life relates in a healthy way with the natural world.

During three decades of collecting stories of indigenous peoples, I have become acquainted with recurring themes that were essential lessons for living in balance. While the natural and cultural references have varied, the message is universal: health and healthy relationships are equated with reciprocity and generosity of spirit. Common truths appear over and over again in oral traditions. In recent years, as codirector of the Stories for Environmental Stewardship Program for the Quebec-Labrador Foundation, I coordinated a network of professionals in environmental education and conservation from Egypt, Israel, Jordan, Lebanon, and Palestine while they gathered narratives from their diverse traditions. Even in a conflict-plagued region such as the Middle East, where countries struggle to find common ground, similar folkloric patterns revealed that there are many shared values relating to family, culture, and environment.

Children possess an inherent belief in the spiritual aspects and connections found among the living and nonliving parts of the earth. Any holistic approach to children, health, and the environment should consider the human spirit as well as the physical. Individuals from a particular culture tend to learn in a distinct way, using the various kinds of human intelligence in unique patterns and combinations. For example, among Native North Americans, and among many other indigenous cultures around the world, traditional education takes the form of initiation rites and direct observation of elders, who hold and pass on important knowledge. Indigenous learning emphasizes certain forms of intelligence, such as spatial, interpersonal, linguistic, and musical.

For example, a common belief among Native North Americans is that human beings are identified with a particular place that defines us, provides for us, and is an inseparable part of who we are. Among the Abenaki of northern New England, the life force embodies emotion, energy, and health. The wellness of a person's spirit depends on the state of his or her mind and the strength of relationships with earth and sky. All life is connected by the healing water, *nebi*, that flows through our veins, replenished and renewed by the land.

In the traditional life of the Abenacki, children would undergo a rite of passage at around age 13. Through fasting and vision seeking, and with the help of an elder guide, young people would look for an ally or helper, a guardian spirit to increase their sense of personal power.

The rituals for boys included a trek to a remote location in the wilds, where they would light a fire and fast. During this time, the youth sang, played songs on his flute, and offered prayers while discovering his true life and the power to move along that journey. The ritual for girls was a time of transition, moving from childhood to becoming a young woman. Her mother, grandmothers, and aunts would build a small moon lodge set apart from the village where the girl, in her visions, sought a guardian spirit of her own to teach and help her through the coming years.

While it is unrealistic to consider creating a modern-day version of the vision quest as a bonding with the natural world—as a transition into adulthood and the onset of a life lived in balance—it is essential that we find a way to help young hearts and minds experience a similar stage of growth and transformation within the context of contemporary life. How do we, in these times, create a social, cultural, educational, and technological context that helps children to live in balance with the natural world? How do we help youth to understand how their own health is interwoven with nature, and to develop a nurturing relationship with plants and animals, soil, water, and sky?

Today a movement known as place-based education uses traditional approaches to teach children about local landscapes, cultures, and social groups. Placed-based education strives to connect youth to local environments and traditions through direct, hands-on community experiences that dovetail with learning through conventional subjects such as science, math, social studies, language, and the arts.

Traveling this road is going to entail a tremendous amount of work because in diverse societies there is no one-size-fits-all approach. But it can be done. We can help children to see their own lives as stories that are unfolding each day, and to realize that they are actively forming the directions of their lives by the kinds of choices they make and actions they decide to take. We can actively encourage an environmental ethic in children by exposing them to the inspiring life stories of such real role models as Rachel Carson, Aldo Leopold, Jane Goodall, John Muir, and the many eco-heroes who are recognized for their great deeds on behalf of the earth.

We can instill in youth the self-confidence to act and believe in the possibility of changing the world for the better. But, finally, we have to continue to work to get children off of their electronic devices and out into the natural world.

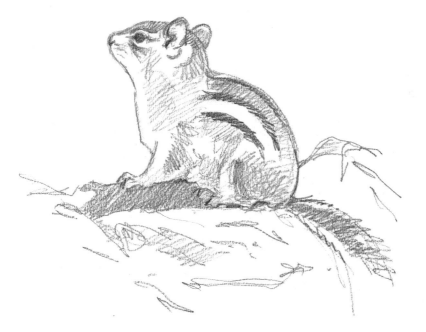

Summer Rain

by Clarisse Hart

In a place with no
dry season, when the ground
cries out for rain: listen—

the dusty rake of the breeze,
the rattle of vacant leaves,

a sprinkler hissing on
to pacify the garden.

Suddenly the air shifts,
sags heavy, like a
two-week balloon.
But it's a promising weight,
not like the dark boxes
you've been carrying.

Hush! What's been
promised for days is now
prickling your skin.

A rush of wind
tousles the coral bells,
and the first drops scatter
down the black rungs
of maidenhair fern,

landing in thick pops
against the dirt.

The sighing ground
steams.

You stand, clothes soaking,
cool rivulets twisting
down your spine.

You set down a few
of the dark boxes.

The beaver, too,
always starts his work
with a flood.

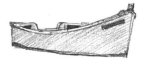

Rhode Island
Quahog Skiff

Wildness and Wellness
by Ann Prince

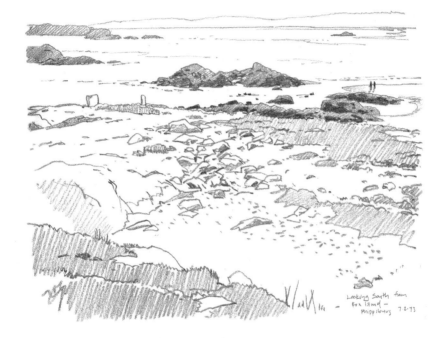

Looking South from
Fox Island —
Phippsburg   7-2-93

Mass Audubon's director of Land Protection, Bob Wilber, has devoted his career to land preservation. He recognizes that every piece of wildland—little or large, close by or faraway—is an asset. Although he's often involved in complex transactions that save large tracts in the state, Wilber, who lives in Stow, knows firsthand that even tiny parcels of green space have great significance. "There's a small place in the woods behind my house where after a long day at work I just sit and relax a little," he says. "The benefits of taking time to decompress in a park or sanctuary are often astonishing."

Mass Audubon owns more than 30,000 acres in our statewide system of wildlife sanctuaries, which represents the largest ownership of privately held land in Massachusetts, in addition to the 5,000 acres the organization holds under conservation restriction. Other permanently protected properties belong to the federal government, the state, municipalities, private organizations, and private citizens.

Over 2,000 square miles—a quarter of the state's land—has been conserved, covering a footprint larger than that of developed land. "Given the fact that Massachusetts is the third most densely populated state in the union," Wilber says, "this is powerful validation of our proud legacy of land conservation."

Ecologically, it is essential to preserve land to keep water pure and drinkable, provide habitat for native wildlife and for plants that release oxygen and consume carbon dioxide, and, in coastal areas, create buffers to compensate for the sea level rise. Not a new concept and equally compelling, conserving land—both wild and tamed—is an asset to health and happiness, for the collective mind, body, and spirit of humanity.

In their essay *The Powerful Link Between Conserving Land and Preserving Human Health*, Howard Frumkin, MD, and Richard Louv demonstrate that time spent absorbed in nature is essential and that land conservation can be considered a strategy for reinforcing public health. In fact, a host of scientific studies are finally documenting what many already knew: human beings have an undeniable need for nature. Yet wilderness and even our planet's atmosphere are severely threatened—the earth is now more vulnerable than ever, and many would argue that our environmental problems stem from an imbalance caused in part by humans' disassociation from the natural world as a result of our industrialized electronic society.

John Cohen, a prominent eco-psychologist, believes that humanity's excesses and overconsumption are directly linked to our lives being separate from the natural environment. "We all make contact through the same planet yet 95 percent of peoples' time is spent indoors," he says. "Our senses are being fulfilled in artificial ways rather than through our inborn attraction to nature."

This trend of separation from our roots in the earth and our branches in the sky has been emerging for a long time. Decades ago, artist Marc Chagall (1887-1985) wrote, "The habit of ignoring nature is deeply implanted in our time. This attitude reminds me of people who never look you in the eye; I find them disturbing and always look away."

Nowadays, when so many distractions work to break our ancestral cord with nature, nevertheless ingrained in every person is an affinity too strong to fully ignore. "There is an inseparable connection between humans and the earth," Wilber says, describing our innate deep-rooted bond with the natural world. This is apparent in adults as well as young children. There is no doubt that communing with nature has a profoundly positive effect.

Children love adventures outdoors. In Scandinavia a reverence for direct nature experience is the cornerstone of education; in fact, there is a Norwegian word, *friluftsliv*, that translates to "free air life." The main tenet of *friluftsliv* is that children must enter into nature in an uncomplicated way, which is their first inclination anyway.

One early-June morning at Mass Audubon's Broad Meadow Brook Wildlife Sanctuary, a group of second graders from West Tatnick Elementary School in Worcester went on a "habitat exploration" with staff naturalist Christy Barnes. The enthusiastic children began with a deluge of questions. "Are there bears?" "Are there porcupines?" "Any turtles?" Once the schoolchildren were satisfied with the answers—no bears, perhaps porcupines, definitely turtles—they followed Christy into the woods, completely captivated by the environment.

Broad Meadow Brook's education coordinator, Elizabeth Lynch, says that there are many things that she admires in young visitors like these. "Their creativity tends to not be stifled," she says. "There's lots of hands-on learning and teaching through inquiry—being in this natural setting leads to that." Next thing the children who've come with their schools become regulars, along with their families. "We have lots of repeaters," says Lynch. "They end up coming back over and over."

That June day in the field, the schoolchildren were unintentionally encountering the intrinsic quality of *friluftsliv*. The group wound along the trail, crossing slow-moving Broad Meadow Brook, listening to melodious birds calling and foghorn-like bullfrogs singing, sniffing skunk cabbage and sassafras leaves, and passing around a crayfish exoskeleton and even a dead dried-up salamander. Although it's a sanctuary of woodlands, wetlands, and meadows, buzzing traffic from Route 20 was loud near the southern boundary: a reminder of the relief afforded all those who wander the five-mile trail system.

All of a sudden one of the girls shuddered—the drama of the day was taking place almost at their feet. A small garter snake was consuming a big green frog. All eyes were on the handsome stripped snake as it unhinged its jaw while the children watched, rapt and now silent, as the reptile continued to swallow. Once the frog had been gulped down whole, the snake slithered away.

The child-nature interface is just one facet when it comes to saving open spaces for people. Adults depend upon green space too. Without oases from the built environment, places to escape from the barrage of electronic messages, according to eco-psychology, we wouldn't have the chance to reorient ourselves with elements of the earth that keep us centered and sane. John Cohen says that our inner attachment to land, water, sky, sun, moon, stars, planets, gravity, wind, rainfall, soil, sown seeds, growth, plants, animals, form, design, color, light, shadow, dawn, nightfall, temperature, all these and more, bring fulfillment and happiness.

The main avenue toward uniting people with nature is preserving land wherever and whenever possible. Every intact piece of the outdoors is a saving grace for someone. Mass Audubon's Bob Wilber states, "I often talk about our land base serving double duty. The peace and solitude that a natural setting provides are increasingly important."

Wilber highlighted some of Mass Audubon's sanctuaries with special attributes—two of which were largely established in the 1970s at opposite corners of the state: High Ledges in northwestern Massachusetts, 15 miles from the Vermont border in the town of Shelburne, and Felix Neck, southeast of Cape Cod in Edgartown on Martha's Vineyard.

According to the principles of eco-psychology, "Reason and language account for only 4 percent of our inherent means to know and love nature."

Martha's Vineyard artist-conservationist Rand Hopkinson is an observer and painter of landscapes. He calls the natural entities, with their magnetic pull that defies words, "the intangibles." At 194-acre Felix Neck, Hopkinson sees the most heart-stopping skies and the most subtle animal signs.

The solitude of this sanctuary is priceless. Across Sengekontacket Pond, beach crowds are omnipresent in midsummer and traffic tirelessly courses along the barrier beach causeway, yet here one can neither see nor hear another human. Hopkinson is philosophical: "The point is the contrast, without being able to come to a quiet place like this your thoughts are always drowned out by the noise. Finding ourselves in the realm of natural events frees us from the day-to-day. We've been caught up in what we thought was important; this reminds us it's not. When you're out on a walk you're able to be more present. What is your awareness? How engaged are you? Why are you here? What are you doing? When you ask yourself the deeper questions, you realize there's this thing going on that's greater than yourself."

Spellbound by the remoteness, visitors to 600-acre High Ledges may believe that the place is enchanted. The songbirds are kindred creatures—hermit thrushes, flutists sounding their heavenly notes in a fern-filled clearing along a wooded wetland; scarlet tanagers, alighting on young slender maples then flying high up into the forest canopy. The color green is ubiquitous—leaves, fronds, grasses, mosses, lichens. Green, "a restful quiet color," according to the Global Healing Center, promotes "soothing harmonious feelings." Blue has a similar effect.

"The blue sky, the brown soil beneath, the grass, the trees, the animals, the wind and rain, and stars are never strange to me," wrote novelist W. H. Hudson (1841-1922), "for I am in and of and am one of them."

Saving open spaces of course extends beyond the boundaries of our small state of Massachusetts. Fortunately, the ongoing movement to conserve millions of acres across the country and around our sphere can help counteract industrial society's indifference to ecology and a sustainable planet.

One federal preserve is the Rachel Carson National Wildlife Refuge—50 miles of Maine coastline that preserves habitat for salt marsh birds, waterfowl, shorebirds, songbirds, and mammals—named in her honor. In 1953 Carson built a summer cottage on Southport Island in the mouth of the Sheepscott River off of Boothbay. As well as writing the seminal environmental book *Silent Spring*, she also wrote *A Sense of Wonder*. The latter book addresses the freshness and instinct that children have for those native things observed out-of-doors that give us breathless joy.

Rachel Carson believed that the wide-eyed excitement for what is beautiful in nature is often dimmed and lost before we become adults. "It is a wholesome and necessary thing," she wrote, "for us to turn again to the earth and in contemplation of her beauties to know the sense of wonder and humility." She herself clearly retained that sense of wonder. It lives on in much of her work. She had "a deep dark woodland" north of her cottage that she called the Lost Woods where she could hear the "hollow boom of the sea striking against the rocks" and watch the migrating monarch butterflies. Carson was instrumental in saving the Lost Woods.

There are public protected areas throughout the country, acquired by government agencies at national, state, regional, and municipal levels. The US National Parks alone comprise more than 400 separate areas covering upwards of 84 million acres. In 2014, 293 million people visited these landmarks, including forests and parks, lakeshores, seashores, and scenic rivers. This does not include national marine sanctuaries (12 million acres), nor the national forests (190 million acres), nor national wildlife refuges (150 million acres).

State parks—some of which are massive in size and comparable in stature and significance to national parks—also draw visitors escaping their overwrought cluttered lifestyles. By 2010 land trust initiatives nationwide had set aside 47 million acres in the US. The Land Trust Alliance, with 1,100 member land trusts from across the country, points out that its goal is to make it possible for every person in America to live within 10 minutes of a park, trail, or green space. Healthfulness for the people served by these places of respite is a primary purpose stated in the organization's comprehensive vision.

Conserving land is essential for humanity all over the globe—and many foreign countries host giant reserves covering thousands of square miles, preserving habitat and wildlife while taking into account the livelihood of local citizens. In sum total there are 160,000 protected areas in the world, covering well over a tenth of the globe's surface, and encompassing both land and sea. The largest national park in the world, 358,000-square-mile Northeast Greenland National Park, is an International Biosphere Reserve. Polar bears, walruses, arctic foxes, and musk oxen are resident mammals. Ptarmigans, great northern divers, snowy owls, and gyrfalcons are among the breeding birds.

Kavango-Zambezi Transfrontier Conservation Area, a protected area made up of properties of the five bordering countries of Angola, Botswana, Namibia, Zambia, and Zimbabwe, covers 111,000 square miles of land and includes 16 national parks. The adjacent nations formed the conservation area through work with the Peace Parks Foundation and the World Fund for Nature with the purpose of allowing migration of mammals across borders and also encouraging tourism. Victoria Falls, a World Heritage Site, is one of the extraordinary features of the area, along with wildlife such as the endangered African elephant, cheetah, and Nile crocodile.

In the 1980s, Mass Audubon formed a partnership to work with conservationists in Belize to establish and sustainably manage parks and reserves. At the time there were already numerous national parks in the country and widespread understanding among Belizeans for the value of their natural heritage. The initial project, working with counterparts in the country, was Programme for Belize (PfB), founded in 1988. The project's principal focus was creation of the Rio Bravo Conservation and Management Area, now amounting to 260,000 acres in the northwestern corner of this small Central American nation.

A tract with tropical forest, pine savannah, wetlands, lagoons, and riparian habitats, Rio Bravo is distinguished by its immense biodiversity, including 400 species of birds, 200 species of trees, and 70 species of mammals. "Thank goodness that the natural beauty of the forests is still ever present and something that can never be improved upon," said PfB Executive Director Edilberto Romero. "Every time of day has a special magic. Morning and evening walks are full of jungle sounds with brilliant flashes of toucans, trogons, parrots, motmots, and the like."

Mass Audubon has continued its longtime relationship with conservationists in Central America through our Belize Conservation Fund and various exchanges, with our naturalists visiting the country to learn and share knowledge as well as playing host to our Belizean friends. In addition to collaborating with Programme for Belize, Mass Audubon also works closely with the Toledo Institute for Development and Environment (TIDE), which works in the southernmost district of the country to help research, monitor, and manage the natural resources there. It was initially formed as a grassroots initiative to respond to manatee poaching, illegal fishing and logging, and destructive farming methods.

Karena Mahung, whose mother, Celia Mahung, is the executive director of TIDE, grew up in Punta Gorda and spent much of her childhood on the cayes of Belize. Her family often took 45-minute weekend boat rides out to the Port Honduras Marine Reserve off the coast from her hometown. "It's a spectacular seascape with an immensely calming effect," she says. "We'd snorkel and swim off West Snake Caye and picnic on a lovely isolated beach. From the tiny mangrove island, in the distance we could see the Guatemalan and Honduran mountainscape. And there were cool wildlife sightings—dolphins, manatees, sea turtles, frigatebirds. The memories of the turqoise blue waters and fishing with my dad bring me a sense of calmness and joy to this day."

"I realize that I am lucky to have parents who had the capacity to provide me with these experiences. The boat trips also allowed me to experience firsthand the realities of illegal fishing by both locals and foreigners in our territorial waters, and poaching of beloved manatees." That is why locals and governmental officials established the reserve in 1997. It protects an array of habitats such as inshore, patch, and fringing reefs; seagrass beds; and 138 mangrove cayes. This invaluable natural resource can now continue to be used sustainably as an important local traditional fishery.

As with other individuals who spent their youth immersed in wilds close to home, Mahung was deeply inspired. "Exposure at a very early age to these natural wonders and the resource management challenges threatening them made me want to be an environmentalist," she adds.

To carry forward her goal to establish a career preserving wildlife, habitats, and local sustainable use of natural resources, Mahung attended the University of the West Indies in Trinidad and Tobago, a regional university for the Caribbean. She majored in Environmental and Resource Management and in 2014 worked as a fall intern at Mass Audubon. Now she's in her second year working on a graduate degree at the Yale School of Forestry and Environmental Studies. She is working toward a career that will focus on ensuring proper management of resources and maintenance of natural areas so that communities that have long cultural and historical ties to the land and sea can continue with their traditional livelihoods. She aims to support innovative conservation finance mechanisms that both increase and maximize investments in conservation, and take preservation much further than acquisition.

The Port Honduras Marine Reserve is a significant resource, especially for the people of Belize. In other parts of the world, some of the largest protected areas are marine reserves. These include the 50-square-mile Galápagos Marine Reserve off the coast of Ecuador, established around a group of islands made famous by scientist Charles Darwin (1809-1882) who voyaged there on *The Beagle* and studied the endemic species. "The love of all creatures," he said, "is the most noble attribute of man." Also renowned is Australia's Great Barrier Reef, which is protected as the centerpiece of a 140,000-square-mile marine park.

"I think that having land and not ruining it is the most beautiful art that anybody could ever want," observed Andy Warhol. The size of a green space, or blue space, really isn't what's important as far as a person's frame of mind is concerned. If not for a pretty backyard, a small urban park, a wild hundred-acre wood, a reserve stretching as far as the eye can see—how can we hear a quiet voice that brings us to a content place within? Nature is our soul.

Epilogue
by A.A. Milne

They walked on, thinking of This and That, and by-and-by they came to an enchanted place on the very top of the Forest called Galleons Lap, which is sixty-something trees in a circle; and Christopher Robin knew that it was enchanted because nobody had ever been able to count whether it was sixty-three or sixty-four, not even when he had tied a piece of string round each tree after he had counted it. Being enchanted, its floor was not like the floor of the Forest, gorse and bracken and heather, but close-set grass, quiet and smooth and green. It was the only place in the Forest where you could sit down carelessly, without getting up again almost at once and looking for somewhere else. Sitting there they could see the whole world spread out until it reached the sky, and whatever there was all the world over was with them in Galleons Lap.

Suddenly Christopher Robin began to tell Pooh about some of the things: People called Kings and Queens and something called Factors, and a place called Europe, and an island in the middle of the sea where no ships came, and how you make a Suction Pump (if you want to), and when Knights were Knighted, and what comes from Brazil. And Pooh, his back against one of the sixty-something trees, and his paws folded in front of him, said "Oh!" and "I didn't know," and thought how wonderful it would be to have a Real Brain which could tell you things. And by-and-by Christopher Robin came to an end of the things, and was silent, and he sat there looking out over the world, and wishing it wouldn't stop.

But Pooh was thinking too, and he said suddenly to Christopher Robin:

"It is a very Grand thing to be an Afternoon, what you said?"

"A what?" said Christopher Robin lazily, as he listened to something else.

"On a horse," explained Pooh.

"A Knight?"

"Oh, was that it?" said Pooh. "I thought it was a—Is it as Grand as a King and Factors and all the other things you said?"

"Well, it's not as grand as a King," said Christopher Robin, and then, as Pooh seemed disappointed, he added quickly, "but it's grander than Factors."

"Could a bear be one?"

"Of course he could!" said Christopher Robin. "I'll make you one." And he took a stick and touched Pooh on the shoulder and said, "Rise, Sir Pooh de Bear, most faithful of all my Knights."

So Pooh rose and sat down and said "Thank you," which is the proper thing to say when you have been made a Knight, and he went into a dream again, in which he and Sir Pomp and Sir Brazil and Factors lived together with a horse, and were faithful Knights, (all except Factors, who looked after the horse) to Good King Christopher Robin…and every now and then he shook his head, and said to himself "I'm not getting it right." Then he began to think of all the things Christopher Robin would want to tell him when he came back from wherever he was going to, and how muddling it would be for a Bear of Very Little Brain to try and get them right in his mind. "So, perhaps," he said sadly to himself, "Christopher Robin won't tell me any more," and he wondered if being a Faithful Knight meant that you just went on being faithful without being told things.

Then, suddenly again, Christopher Robin, who was still looking at the world, with his chin in his hands, called out "Pooh!"

"Yes?" said Pooh.

"When I'm—when—Pooh!"

"Yes, Christopher Robin?"

"I'm not going to do Nothing any more."

"Never again?"

"Well, not so much. They don't let you."

Pooh waited for him to go on, but he was silent again.

"Yes, Christopher Robin?" said Pooh helpfully.

"Pooh, when I'm—you know—when I'm *not* doing Nothing, will you come up here sometimes?"

"Just me?"

"Yes, Pooh."

"Will you be here too?"

"Yes, Pooh, I will be, *really*. I *promise* I will be, Pooh."

"That's good," said Pooh.

"Pooh, *promise* you won't forget about me, ever. Not even when I'm a hundred."

Pooh thought for a little.

"How old shall *I* be then?"

"Ninety-nine."

Pooh nodded.

"I promise," he said.

Still with his eyes on the world, Christopher Robin put out a hand and felt for Pooh's paw.

"Pooh," said Christopher Robin, earnestly, "if I—if I'm not quite—" he stopped and tried again—"Pooh, *whatever* happens, you *will* understand, won't you?"

"Understand what?"

"Oh, nothing." He laughed and jumped to his feet. "Come on!"

"Where?" said Pooh.

"Anywhere," said Christopher Robin.

So they went off together. But wherever they go, and whatever happens to them on the way, in that enchanted place on the top of the Forest, a little boy and his Bear will always be playing.

The House at Pooh Corner by A. A. Milne, copyright © 1956, A. A. Milne. All rights reserved.

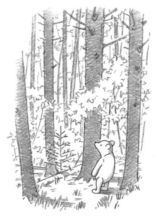

Poet Biographies

Brad Bennett's haiku have appeared in over twenty print and online publications. His favorite Mass Audubon sanctuaries are Broadmoor and Ipswich River.

Polly Brown, of Every Other Thursday Poets, has written about war and peace through the Joiner Institute at UMass Boston, and organized plein air poetry in Hopkinton.

Wendy Drexler's poems have appeared in *Mid-American Review, Nimrod, Prairie Schooner*, and others. She is a three-time Pushcart Prize nominee and author of a book-length collection, *Western Motel*.

Sarah Goodman is coauthor of *Ferry Ride*. She exhibited a matchbox photo book, *Seven Deadly Verses*.

Holly Guran is author of *River of Bones* and the chapbooks *River Tracks* and *Mothers' Trails*.

Jeffrey Harrison's fifth book of poetry, *Into Daylight*, was published by Tupelo Press in 2014 as winner of the Dorset Prize.

Clarisse Hart is outreach and development manager for education and research programs at Harvard Forest in Petersham, Massachusetts. Her work has appeared in *Orion* and *Ecotone*.

Jack Kerouac was an American novelist and poet, and a pioneer of the Beat Generation.

Frannie Lindsay's work appeared in *Best American Poetry 2014*. Her books of poetry are *Our Vanishing, Mayweed, Lamb, Where She Always Was,* and *If Mercy*.

Moira Lineman is author of *If No Moon* and *Incarnate Grace*.

Christopher Locke is the nonfiction editor of *Slice* magazine. His collection of travel poems and essays, *Ordinary Gods*, is forthcoming in 2017.

Kathy Nelson is the author of *Cattails*. Her poems have appeared in *U.S. 1 Worksheets, Off the Coast, The Cortland Review, Switched-on Gutenberg,* and *Paterson Literary Review*.

Susan Edwards Richmond is poet-in-residence at *Old Frog Pond Farm & Studio*. She is the author of four poetry collections, *Increase, Birding in Winter, Purgatory Chasm,* and *Boto*.

Sophie Wadsworth is the executive director of The Nature Connection in Concord, Massachusetts. She is the author of *Letters from Siberia*, winner of the Jessie Bryce Niles Chapbook Award.

Margot Wizansky has been published in *Poetry East, Lumina,* and *Tar River Poetry*. In 2010, she won the Patricia Dobler Poetry Award to study in Ireland.

Writer Biographies

Nini Bloch is a writer who covers field science, environmental topics, and animal behavior.

Michael J. Caduto devotes his time to teaching children and adults about nature and earth stewardship. He travels the world as an ecologist, educator, storyteller, and award-winning author. His website is www.p-e-a-c-e.net.

Teri Dunn Chace is a garden writer. Her latest book is *Seeing Seeds: A Journey into the World of Seedheads, Pods, and Fruit* (2015).

Thomas Conuel teaches journalism and is the author of *Quabbin: The Accidental Wilderness* and coauthor of *The Nature of Massachusetts*.

Gayle Goddard-Taylor is a freelance journalist who specializes in animals and the environment.

Ron McAdow is the former executive director of the Sudbury Valley Trustees and author of guidebooks to the Concord and Charles rivers and the novel *Ike*.

John Hanson Mitchell was the editor of Mass Audubon's journal, *Sanctuary*, and author of six books about a single square mile of land, collected together as The Scratch Flat Chronicles.

Karl Meyer is an award-winning book author and a member of the Society of Environmental Jounalists. His River Report is heard Tuesdays on WHMP radio. www.karlmeyerwriting.com/blog.

Ann Prince is a staff writer-editor for Mass Audubon, and a naturalist, artist, and mother of three.

Artist Biography

Barry W. Van Dusen is an internationally recognized wildlife artist living in central Massachusetts. His work has appeared in books published by the American Birding Association, HarperCollins, Princeton University Press, and Cornell University (Comstock). His paintings have been featured in *Bird Watcher's Digest, Birder's World, Birds Illustrated (U.K.), Wildlife Art,* and *Yankee* magazines. Barry is currently artist in residence for Mass Audubon's Museum of American Bird Art (MABA). He is traveling the state chronicling through his artwork the rich and diverse landscapes, habitats, and animal life at our 56 wildlife sanctuaries. His residency will culminate with an exhibition at MABA in 2017.